PLANS OF CARE FOR SPECIALTY PRACTICE

Orthopaedic Nursing

LEONA MOURAD, MS, RN, ONC
Nursing Consultant
Mourad Consultant Associates
Columbus, Ohio

series editor
KATHY V. GETTRUST, RN, BSN
Case Manager
Midwest Medical Home Care
Milwaukee, Wisconsin

Delmar Publishers Inc.™

ITP™ An International Thomson Publishing Company

**New York • London • Bonn • Boston • Detroit • Madrid • Melbourne • Mexico City • Paris
Singapore • Tokyo • Toronto • Washington • Albany NY • Belmont CA • Cincinnati OH**

NOTICE TO THE READER

Publisher does not warrant or guarantee any of the products described herein or perform any independent analysis in connection with any of the product information contained herein. Publisher does not assume, and expressly disclaims, any obligation to obtain and include information other than that provided to it by the manufacturer.

The reader is expressly warned to consider and adopt all safety precautions that might be indicated by the activities described herein and to avoid all potential hazards. By following the instructions contained herein, the reader willingly assumes all risks in connection with such instructions.

The publisher makes no representations or warranties of any kind, including but not limited to, the warranties of fitness for particular purpose or merchantability, nor are any such representations implied with respect to the material set forth herein, and the publisher takes no responsibility with respect to such material. The publisher shall not be liable for any special, consequential or exemplary damages resulting, in whole or in part, from the readers' use of, or reliance upon, this material.

Cover Illustration: Jeanne Benas

Delmar Staff
Publisher: David C. Gordon
Acquisitions Editor: Patricia E. Casey
Associate Editor: Elisabeth F. Williams
Project Editor: Danya M. Plotsky
Production Coordinator: Barbara A. Bullock
Art and Design Coordinator: Mary E. Siener
Editorial Assistant: Tonjia Herman

Printed in the United States of America

For more information, contact:

Delmar Publishers Inc.
3 Columbia Circle, Box 15015
Albany, NY 12212-5015

International Thomson Publishing
Berkshire House
168-173 High Holborn
London, WC1V7AA
England

Thomas Nelson Australia
102 Dodds Street
South Melbourne 3205
Victoria, Australia

Nelson Canada
1120 Birchmont Road
Scarborough, Ontario
M1K 5G4, Canada

International Thomson Publishing GmbH
Konigswinterer Str. 418
53227 Bonn
Germany

International Thomson Publishing Asia
221 Henderson Bldg. #05-10
Singapore 0315

International Thomson Publishing Japan
Kyowa Building, 3F
2-2-1 Hirakawa-cho
Chiyoda-ku, Tokyo 102
Japan

1 2 3 4 5 6 7 8 9 10 XXX 00 99 98 97 96 95 94

Library of Congress Cataloging-in-Publication Data

Mourad, Leona A.
Orthopaedic nursing / Leona Mourad
p. cm. — (Plans of care for specialty practice)
Includes bibliographical references and index.
ISBN 0-8273-5944-6
1. Orthopaedic nursing. 2. Nursing care plans. I. Title. II. Series.
RD753.M693 1994
610.73—dc20

94-16955
CIP

TABLE OF CONTENTS

PREFACE

Nursing care of the patient with orthopaedic injuries is complex because of the acuteness or severity of the injuries, the technological equipment, and at times, the multiple organ involvement. Nurses caring for these patients must apply current principles, concepts, and facts for optimal care using the nursing process.

This series of books has been developed to provide a standard for nursing care for all patients. Through the nursing process, care plans provide individualized care specific to the patients discussed in each book.

This book on orthopaedic care plans in the nursing process provides the bases for patients with the most frequently encountered conditions. Chapters are devoted to nursing diagnoses and care plans for patients with musculoskeletal trauma (including fractures and their various treatments), degenerative and inflammatory conditions, metabolic diseases of bones, infections, bone and bone marrow tumors, surgical procedures including total joint replacements, ligament and meniscal repairs, and limb-lengthening procedures. Spinal conditions are discussed with appropriate nursing diagnoses and care plans. Lastly, commonly occurring complications are discussed. Rationales are given for all nursing interventions, and discharge planning and community care factors are also included.

It is hoped that the content and nursing care plans incorporated in this book will be pertinent and indispensable to nurses caring for orthopaedic patients. It has been written with these goals in mind.

Leona A. Mourad
Columbus, Ohio

ACKNOWLEDGMENTS

I want to thank Connie Prouty and Florence Searfoss, whose skills in word processing made the speedy completion of this manuscript possible. They were a pleasure to work with and made the process an easier one.

I also greatly appreciate all the guidance, suggestions, and skilled editing of Beth Williams of Delmar Publishers, Inc.

Finally, I am grateful to my husband, George, who continues to support me through my writing efforts.

Leona Mourad

SERIES INTRODUCTION

Scientific and technological developments over the past several decades have revolutionized health care and care of the sick. These rapid and extensive advancements of knowledge have occurred in all fields, necessitating an ever-increasing specialization of practice. For nurses to be effective and meet the challenge in today's specialty settings, the body of clinical knowledge and skill needs to continually expand. *Plans of Care for Specialty Practice* has been written to aid the practicing nurse in meeting this challenge. The purpose of this series is to provide comprehensive, state-of-the-art plans of care and associated resource information for patient situations most commonly seen within a specialty that will serve as a standard from which care can be individualized. These plans of care are based on the profession's scientific approach to problem solving—the nursing process. Though the books are primarily written as a guide for frontline staff nurses and clinical nurse specialists practicing in specialty settings, they have application for nursing students as well.

DOCUMENTATION OF CARE

The Joint Commission on Accreditation of Healthcare Organizations (JCAHO) assumes authority for evaluating the quality and effectiveness of the practice of nursing. In 1991, the JCAHO developed its first new nursing care standards in more than a decade. One of the changes brought about by these new standards was the elimination of need for every patient to have a handwritten or computer-generated care plan in his or her chart detailing all or most of the care to be provided. The Joint Commission's standard that describes the documentation requirements stipulates that nursing assessments, identification of nursing diagnoses and/or patient care needs, interventions, outcomes of care, and discharge planning be permanently integrated into the clinical record. In other words, the nursing process needs to be documented. A separate care plan is no longer needed; however, planning and implementing care must continue as always, but using whatever form of documentation that has been approved by an institution. *Plans of Care for Specialty Practice* can be easily used with a wide variety of approaches to documentation of care.

ELEMENTS OF THE PLANS OF CARE

The chapter title is the presenting situation, which represents the most commonly seen conditions/disorders treated within the specialty setting. It may be a medical diagnosis (e.g., diabetes mellitis), a syndrome (e.g., acquired immunodeficiency syndrome), a surgical procedure (e.g., mastectomy), or a diagnostic/therapeutic procedure (e.g., thrombolytic therapy).

An opening paragraph provides a definition or concise overview of the presenting situation. It describes the condition and may contain pertinent physiologic/psychologic bases for the disorder. It is brief and not intended to replace further investigation for comprehensive understanding of the condition.

Etiologies

A listing of causative factors responsible for or contributing to the presenting situation is provided. This may include predisposing diseases, injuries or trauma, surgeries, microorganisms, genetic factors, environmental hazards, drugs, or psychosocial disorders. In presenting situations where no clear causal relationship can be established, current theories regarding the etiology may be included.

Clinical Manifestations

Objective and subjective signs and symptoms that describe the particular presenting situation are included. This information is revealed as a result of a health history and physical assessment and becomes part of the data base.

Clinical/Diagnostic Findings

This component contains possible diagnostic tests and procedures that might be done to determine abnormalities associated with a particular presenting situation. The name of the diagnostic procedure and the usual abnormal findings are listed.

Nursing Diagnosis

The nursing management of the health problem commences with the planning care phase of the nursing process. This includes obtaining a comprehensive history and physical assessment, identification of the nursing diagnoses, expected outcomes, interventions, and discharge planning needs.

Diagnostic labels identified by NANDA through the Tenth National Conference in April 1992 are being used throughout this series. (Based on North American Nursing Diagnosis Association, 1992. *NANDA Nursing Diagnoses: Definitions and Classification 1992–1993,* Philadelphia: NANDA.) We have also identified new diagnoses not yet on the official NANDA list. We endorse NANDA's recommendation for nurses to develop new nursing diagnoses as the need arises and we encourage nurses using this series to do the same.

"Related To" Statements

"Related to" statements suggest a link or connection to the nursing diagnosis and provide direction for identifying appropriate nursing interventions. They have sometimes been termed contributing factors, causes, or etiologies. There is frequently more than one "related to" statement for a given diagnosis. For example, change in job, marital difficulties, and impending surgery may all be "related to" the patient's nursing diagnosis of "Anxiety."

There is disagreement at present regarding inclusion of pathophysiologic/medical diagnoses in the list of "related to" statements. Frequently, a medical diagnosis does not provide adequate direction for nursing care. For example, the nursing diagnosis of "Chronic Pain" related to rheumatoid arthritis does not readily suggest specific nursing interventions. It is more useful for the nurse to identify specific causes of the chronic pain, such as inflammation, swelling, and fatigue; these in turn suggest more specific interventions. In cases where the medical diagnosis provides the best available information, as occurs with the more medically oriented diagnoses such as "Decreased Cardiac Output" or "Impaired Gas Exchange," the medical terminology is included.

Defining Characteristics

Data collection is frequently the source for identifying defining characteristics, sometimes called signs and symptoms or patient behaviors. These data, both subjective and objective, are organized into meaningful patterns and used to verify the nursing diagnosis. The most commonly seen defining characteristics for a given diagnosis are included and should not be viewed as an all-inclusive listing.

Risk Factors

Nursing diagnoses designated as high risk are supported by risk factors that direct nursing actions to reduce or prevent the problem from developing. Since these nursing diagnoses have not yet occurred, risk factors replace the listing of actual defining characteristics and "related to" statements.

Patient Outcomes

Patient outcomes, sometimes termed patient goals, are observable behaviors or data that measure changes in the condition of the patient after nursing treatment. They are objective indicators of progress toward prevention of the development of high-risk nursing diagnoses or resolution/modification of actual diagnoses. Like other elements of the plan of care, patient outcome statements are dynamic and must be reviewed and modified periodically as the patient progresses. Assigning realistic "target or evaluation dates" for evaluation of progress toward outcome achievement is crucial. Since there are so many considerations involved in when the outcome could be achieved (e.g., varying lengths of stay, individual patient condition), these plans of care do not include evaluation dates; the date needs to be individualized and assigned using the professional judgment and discretion of the nurse caring for the patient.

Nursing Interventions

Nursing interventions are the treatment options/actions the nurse employs to prevent, modify, or resolve the nursing diagnosis. They are driven by the "related to" statements and risk factors and are selected based on the outcomes to be achieved. Treatment options should be chosen only if they apply realistically to a specific patient condition. The nurse also needs to determine frequencies for each intervention based on professional judgment and individual patient need.

We have included independent, interdependent, and dependent nursing interventions as they reflect current practice. We have not made a distinction between these kinds of interventions because of institutional differences and increasing independence in nursing practice. The interventions that are interdependent or dependent will require collaboration with other professionals. The nurse will need to determine when this is necessary and take appropriate action. The interventions include assessment, therapeutic, and teaching actions.

Rationales

The rationales provide scientific explanations or theoretical bases for the intervention; interventions can then be selected more intelligently and actions can be tailored to each individual's needs.

The rationales provided may be used as a quick reference for the nurse unfamiliar with the reason for a given intervention and as a tool for patient education. These rationales may include principles, theory, and/or research findings from current literature. The rationales are intended as reference information and, as such, should not be transcribed into the permanent patient record. A rationale is not provided when the intervention is self-explanatory.

Discharge Planning/Continuity of Care

Because stays in acute care hospitals are becoming shorter due to cost-containment efforts, patients are frequently discharged still needing care; discharge planning is the process of anticipating and planning for needs after discharge. Effective discharge planning begins with admission and continues with ongoing assessment of the patient and family needs. Included in the discharge planning/continuity of care section are suggestions for follow-up measures, such as skilled nursing care; physical, occupational, speech, or psychiatric therapy; spiritual counseling; social service assistance; follow-up appointments; and equipment/supplies.

References

A listing of references appears at the conclusion of each plan of care or related group of plans. The purpose of the references is to cite specific work used and to specify background information or suggestions for further reading. Citings provided represent the most current nursing theory and/or research bases for inclusion in the plans of care.

Clinical Clips

Interspersed throughout the books are brief pieces of information related to the particular specialty. The intent is to blend some concept or theory tidbits with the practical nature of the books. This information not only may enrich the nurse's knowledge base but also may be used in the dissemination of patient education information.

A WORD ABOUT FAMILY

The authors and editors of this series recognize the vital role that family and/or other significant people play in the recovery of a patient. Isolation from the family unit during hospitalization may disrupt self-concept and feelings of security. Family members, or persons involved in the patient's care, must be included in the teaching to ensure that it is appropriate and will be followed. In an effort to constrain the book's size, the patient outcome, nursing intervention, and discharge planning sections usually do not include reference to the family or other significant people; however, the reader can assume that they are to be included along with the patient whenever appropriate.

ACKNOWLEDGMENTS

Any undertaking of the magnitude of this series becomes the concern of many people. I would specifically like to thank all of the very capable nursing specialists who authored or edited the individual books. Their attention to providing state-of-the-art information in a quick, usable form will provide the reader with current reference information for providing excellent patient care.

Special thanks also goes to my friend Mark Gregory for his clever coinage of the term "clinical clips."

The editorial staff, particularly Patricia E. Casey and Elisabeth F. Williams, and production people at Delmar Publishers have been outstanding. Their frank criticism, comments, and encouragement have improved the quality of the series.

Finally, but most importantly, I wish to thank my husband, John, and children, Katrina and Allison, for their sacrifices and patience during yet another publishing project.

Kathy V. Gettrust
Series Editor

LIST OF TABLES

Musculoskeletal Trauma

Musculoskeletal trauma is a major cause of loss of one's usual roles and activities and economic losses and a frequent cause of death in persons under 40 years of age. More than 150,000 persons die from trauma yearly, with nearly 3.7 million persons hospitalized for treatments of injuries. Common causes of deaths are head injuries related to automobile, motorcycle, or pedestrian accidents. Nonfatal injuries may range from minor injuries such as contusions, sprains, strains, dislocations or subluxations, with one or more fractures being more severe, or major injuries. Definitions, causes, and treatments of various types of minor injuries are shown in Table 1.1, page 17.

FRACTURES

A fracture is a break in one or more cortices of a bone. A fracture may be *closed* if the skin is intact or *open* if the skin is disrupted at the site; it may be across a bone (transverse), vertically or obliquely across a bone (spiral or oblique), more than two fragments (comminuted), or squeezed together on one side (compressed). It may be out of its usual anatomic position (displaced, angulated) or within (intra-articular) or outside (extra-articular) a joint (see Table 1.2, page 18).

Frequently there is soft tissue injury associated with a fracture leading to bleeding, swelling, discoloration, loss of feeling or numbness, and loss of function. The fracture site is also cooler. Inflammatory changes occur at the fracture site to bring about bone healing, as shown in Table 1.3, page 19.

ETIOLOGIES

- Accident leading to fracture(s)
- Fall on affected part
- Moderate to severe blow to site
- Weakened area in bone from tumor or lack of proper vitamins or minerals, especially calcium
- Gun shot wound to bone and surrounding tissues

CLINICAL MANIFESTATIONS

- Coolness at site
- Inability to use affected part normally
- Presence of swelling, numbness or pain, color changes

CLINICAL/DIAGNOSTIC FINDINGS

- Physical examination shows manifestations given above.
- History elicits accident, gun shot wound, fall, or blow to part; may have history of low calcium intake.

- Roentgenogram, computerized tomography (CT), or magnetic resonance imaging (MRI) shows discontinuity in one or more cortices of one or more bones or presence of tumor.
- Hematologic studies may show low calcium levels.

▶ NURSING DIAGNOSIS: *Impaired Physical Mobility*

Related To presence of fracture(s) and soft tissue trauma

Defining Characteristics

- Inability to use part normally
- Presence of tumor in one or more areas of body
- Weakened or deformed bones

Patient Outcomes

The patient will

- regain bone continuity after treatments and healing time.
- retain muscle/joint functions in unaffected tissues.
- regain usual mobility after bone healing and treatments.

Nursing Interventions	Rationales
Assess site(s) for signs of bleeding, edema, color changes, pain, numbness or tingling, and inability to use part.	Assessment and determining degrees of deviation from normal give data of severity of injury.
Position person as comfortably as possible; may use pillows to aid in positioning or elevation; handle tissues gently.	Patient may have difficulty maintaining proper positions because of injuries or pain. Pillows aid maintenance of proper positions and elevation. Elevation lessens development of edema. Bedrest may be required as part of treatments.
Perform all neurovascular checks as per physician's prescription.	Neurovascular data provide evidence of ongoing conditions in affected part. **See Table 1.4, page 21, for steps and rationale of neurovascular checks.**
Assist with definitive treatment: may have application of skin or skeletal traction (Table 1.5, page 22), cast, external fixator (Table 1.6, page 27), or cast brace.	Specific treatment(s) vary according to the particular injury, site, age of patient, or other pertinent patient conditions.
Apply ice to affected part.	Ice lessens bleeding, edema, and pain.

▶ NURSING DIAGNOSIS: *Acute Pain*

Related To fracture(s) and soft tissue trauma

Defining Characteristics

- Angulation of fracture fragments
- Expresses pain if injured parts are moved
- Presence of break in one or more bones
- Protective of affected tissues
- Restless, anxious, or fearful
- Rubbing of broken ends against each other or contiguous tissues
- Vital sign changes: may be increases or decreases in temperature, blood pressure, pulse, or respirations
- Wincing, grimacing, moaning, or crying

Patient Outcomes

The patient will

- experience relief of pain with treatments and healing.
- express relief of pain after medication administration and absorption.
- rarely exhibit behaviors associated with pain such as only occasional winces, moans, or grimaces with use of affected parts.

Nursing Interventions	Rationales
Assess for characteristics of pain: type, sites, duration, severity, patterns, precipitating or alleviating factors.	Individuals have personal responses to pain; their behaviors must be thoroughly assessed and appropriately responded to as determined from the data.
Discuss use of pain-alleviating activities with patient and willingness to use such methods.	Pain may be eased with changes in positions, use of ice applications, massage to uninjured tissues, relaxation techniques, specific exercises, elevation of injured parts, or administration of medications.
Implement patient's choice for pain relief measure(s).	Patient may choose one or more measures, alone or along with medications.
Administer narcotic or nonnarcotic analgesic as prescribed. Patient may be using patient-controlled analgesia (PCA).	Patient-controlled analgesia allows patient to have more personal control over pain relief. If PCA not in use, nurses should initially administer analgesics

Nursing Interventions	Rationales
	around the clock to help maintain therapeutic blood levels.
If prescribed, administer anti-inflammatory medications between narcotic dosages.	Anti-inflammatory medications enhance pain relief by increasing resolution of inflammation in injury sites.
Teach patient use of stress reduction techniques, relaxation techniques, imagery, or music, if desired.	Each of these activities provides muscle relaxation which increases circulation, aids in removing inflammatory wastes, and increases patient's control of painful episodes.
Use distraction techniques when appropriate; these techniques may include games, cards, humor, reading aloud, or selected group activities such as singing.	Distraction helps patient focus outwardly and temporarily away from the pain situation.

NOTE: See page 283 for discussion of chronic pain related to fractures.

▶ NURSING DIAGNOSIS: *Altered Tissue Perfusion*

Related To fracture and soft tissue injury

Defining Characteristics

- Complaints of numbness, tingling, or frank pain
- Coolness of affected tissues
- Discontinuity in bone(s) with angulation and displacement
- Presence of edema, color changes, and bruising

Patient Outcomes

The patient will

- experience no complications related to fracture injuries or altered healing.
- regain usual (normal) tissue integrity and perfusion following treatments and healing.

Nursing Interventions	Rationales
Assess site(s) of injuries for neurovascular functions.	See Table 1.4, page 21, for all steps and rationales for neurovascular checks.
Apply ice to sites.	Ice constricts capillaries, decreases bleeding, and lessens edema formation. RICE = Rest, Ice, Compression, Elevation.
Elevate injured tissues on pillow or pillows.	Elevation aids venous return to lessen edema formation.
Reposition patient q2–4h.	Repositioning avoids excessive pressure on dependent tissues.
If edema is pronounced, initiate activities to monitor compartment pressures.	See page 299 for discussion of compartment syndrome.
Monitor hematocrit and hemoglobin data daily.	Bleeding (or hemorrhage) may be marked depending on the site or fractures, as, e.g., following a fracture of the hip, the patient may bleed up to 1,000 mL into the joint area.
Observe injury site daily for evidence of resolution of inflammation and/or infection.	Following an injury and fracture, the affected tissues go through inflammatory changes (see Table 1.3, page 19). Infection is a possibility if the skin is broken from either outside in or inside out, as in an open fracture.
Prepare the patient for the selected definitive treatment after physician, patient, and family discussions and diagnostic tests.	The physician determines the most likely injuries after securing a history, doing a physical examination, and diagnostic tests including hematologic, cardiovascular, and roentgenographic studies. The physician discusses proposed treatments with the family and patient for mutual goal setting.
Assist with the selected definitive treatment as appropriate.	Definitive treatments may include application of a splint, brace, cast, external fixator, traction, or surgical correction and internal fixation. See the index for the page for each treatment's discussion.

▶ NURSING DIAGNOSIS: *Impaired Gas Exchange*

Related To spinal, thoracic, or upper extremity fractures and/or soft tissue injuries

Defining Characteristics

- Bleeding and bruising into or around fracture sites
- Bedrest with skull tong traction if cervical vertebral fracture
- Hesitation to take deep breaths with fractured ribs
- Injury to lung tissues with fractured ribs
- Potential for fat or pulmonary embolism with long-bone (humerus) fracture
- Potential for nerve injury with vertebral or humeral fractures
- Presence of one or more fractures of humerus, ribs, or vertebra

Patient Outcomes

The patient will

- experience no pulmonary complications such as fat or pulmonary embolism or pneumonia.
- have clear breath sounds in all lobes.
- regain eupneic status after treatments.
- retain as much normally functioning pulmonary tissues during treatments and fracture healing.

Nursing Interventions	Rationales
Assess for breath sounds, rales, or rhonchi in all lobes.	Breath sounds should be heard clearly in all lobes. Rales and rhonchi are adventitious sounds indicative of presence of secretions in respiratory passages.
Assess respiratory functions with vital signs; note any hesitation or gasping for breath, holding breath, or increased, irregular, or shallow respirations.	Respiratory rates may be increased, irregular, or shallow due to pain, presence of rib fractures, lung trauma, fear, or anxiety. Hesitation may occur due to fractured bones rubbing against each other. Holding the breath may occur due to pain, faulty nerve transmission, or fear. Respiratory rates may be increased due to anemia or blood loss from hemorrhage.

Nursing Interventions	Rationales
Monitor for color changes in lips, nail beds, or skin.	Hypoxia and anoxia may be noted by bluish color of lips and nail beds and paleness or bluish skin tinges.
Listen to patient's complaints of sudden pain in chest, changes in vital signs (increases in pulse and respirations, altered blood pressure), sense of dread or doom, anxiety, development of dyspnea, disorientation, confusion, change in mental alertness, pallor, cyanosis, and development of a fine, petechial rash from nipple line on chest up to neck and on eyelids or conjunctivae.	The symptoms listed are commonly seen in fat emboli which most commonly occur 1–3 days after a long-bone fracture. See page 315 for thorough discussion of fat and pulmonary emboli which occur 10–12 days after trauma and secondary to thrombophlebitis. Fat emboli impair gas exchange and must be treated quickly and vigorously to prevent death.
Perform Homan sign by dorsiflexing patient's feet, one at a time.	Presence of dull or sharp pain deep in the calf while the foot is dorsiflexed is a positive Homan sign and is one indication of thrombophlebitis. An embolism from such a site may break loose, travel to the lung, and block passage of gases through lungs, thereby impairing gas exchange.
Encourage patient to do deep-breathing exercises and to use incentive spirometer, if prescribed, q2h.	Deep-breathing exercises enhance lung expansion and aid in gas exchange. A patient with fractured ribs may be unable to use an incentive spirometer until some healing has occurred.
Monitor cough, if present; check sputum for color and amount.	Presence of a cough with productive, yellow or green sputum may signify development of pneumonia.
Assist patient to alter positions q2h, if able to be moved. If on a special bed, such as CircOlectric, rotate anterior and posterior frames q2–3h.	Altering or changing positions increases circulation to dependent areas, lessens chance of development of pressure areas, and aids gas exchange.
If trauma is such that the patient may be up, assist to ambulate q4h, if able.	Ambulation aids healing and gas exchange and lessens risk of thrombophlebitis.

▶ NURSING DIAGNOSIS: *High Risk for Disuse Syndrome*

Risk Factors

- Imposed bedrest
- Fractures of skeletal bones of spine, ribs, and humerus
- Decreased ennervation from nerve trauma
- Decreased motor functions from vertebral trauma
- Weakness or paralysis of muscles
- Decreased muscle mass

Patient Outcomes

The patient will

- experience no permanent nerve/muscle deficits.
- regain as much function as possible with treatments.
- participate as actively as possible in rehabilitation activities.
- maintain as much nerve/muscle functions as possible.

Nursing Interventions	Rationales
Assess all muscles and joints for functions and range of motion (ROM).	Assessments provide data of extent of the injuries and possible needed treatments to restore functions.
Assess condition of the skin, bony prominences, and need for special beds, mattresses, or pressure reduction devices.	Assessments help determine patient's condition and special needs.
Provide active and passive ROM exercises to uninjured muscles and joints.	Exercises increase circulation, distribution of nutrients, and removal of wastes to help maintain strength in muscles and joints.
Consult with physical/occupational therapists as needed.	Specific health team members provide specialized services to aid patient's recovery.
Reposition patient q2h.	Repositioning lessens pressure on dependent tissues and bony prominences to prevent development of pressure areas.
Provide skin care several times daily; check skin areas for moistness or dry areas; keep bed linens dry and wrinkle free.	Skin care increases circulation to remove wastes. Skin should be kept dry to prevent maceration. Wrinkle-free linens decrease pressure spots or areas.

Nursing Interventions	Rationales
Provide splints, foot supports, braces, or immobilizers, if needed.	Supports help weak or paralyzed muscles maintain alignment to prevent contractures.
Provide isometric or isotonic exercises as needed.	These exercises prevent stasis, thus lessening possibility of development of thrombophlebitis.
Encourage deep-breathing exercises, as able; use special respiratory treatments such as intermittent positive pressure breathing (IPPB).	Bedrest limits respiratory functions, as do rib fractures. Special respiratory therapies may be needed to prevent pulmonary infections.
Consult with dietitian for high-nutrient diet; provide fluid intake q2h.	Patients on bed rest may lose weight and muscle mass. They need a high-vitamin and high-protein diet, plus 3,000 mL fluid daily to restore nutrient and fluid balances. Foods should be high in fiber to maintain proper bowel elimination.
Encourage patient and family members to learn self-care and application of splints or braces within patient's limitations and needs.	Being able to participate in care provides positive motivation toward recovery.
Teach patient and family members limitations and safe care related to use of assistive devices, cast, brace, or traction.	Learning safe care techniques provides for continuity of care.

▶ NURSING DIAGNOSIS: *Knowledge Deficit*

Related To unexpected trauma, fractures, and types of deficits (if present), and proposed treatments.

Defining Characteristics

- Angulated, displaced fracture of humerus
- Anterior fractures of ribs 7 and 8
- Application of halo traction and cast
- Cervical traction with skull tongs (possible)
- Discussion of multiple proposed treatments with unfamiliar terms

- Presence of paresis/paralysis
- Presence of one or more fractures of vertebrae, ribs, or humerus
- Suddenness and severity of trauma

Patient Outcomes

The patient will
- participate in discussion of condition and treatments as condition permits, alone or with family members.
- understand terms used during discussions.
- participate in goal setting and treatment regimen as able.
- learn self-care techniques within limitations of condition.

Nursing Interventions	Rationales
Assess patient's/family's understanding of physician's explanations.	Data are vital for teaching of patient and family.
Clarify patient's questions related to condition or proposed treatments.	Repeated explanations may be needed because of patient's condition, newness or unfamiliarity with terms, fear or anxiety, or other reasons.
Use diagrams, pictures, or charts when discussing treatments with patient or family.	Various methods may be needed for best learning experiences.
Identify self-care or home care needs according to patient's injuries, treatments, and ability to learn and do self-care.	Identification of self-care needs is an initial step in learning and teaching care.
Teach patient/family members self or home care needs.	Several sessions may be needed for learning specific aspects of care, such as cast care, use of walker or crutches, pin care with external fixator, or wound care.
Identify personnel and resources available to patient when discharged.	Family members/significant others, social services or financial aid, plus rehabilitation equipment or personnel such as physical or occupational therapists may be needed.
Provide written instructions for self-care at home.	Having written instructions is a safety factor as well as provides a

Nursing Interventions	Rationales
	measure of security for patient/family/significant other.
Evaluate patient's readiness for self-care and discharge by observing care over time.	The patient may require a period of time to learn own care due to his or her condition, ability to learn, or complexity of care requirements.

▶ NURSING DIAGNOSIS: *Self-Care Deficit—Bathing/Hygiene*

Related To fractured humerus with internal fixation compression plate and screws

Defining Characteristics

- Angulated, displaced fracture of right humerus
- Inability to use right arm and forearm both preoperatively and for a period of time postoperatively
- Is right handed
- Presence of fractures of number 7 and 8 ribs

Patient Outcomes

The patient will

- learn to use left hand and left upper extremity to do bathing and hygiene after surgical correction and while wound heals.
- regain use of right hand and upper extremity after fracture treatment and fracture and wound healing.

Nursing Interventions	Rationales
Assess patient's ability to use left hand/upper extremity to assist with bath and hygiene.	Patient's overall condition and fractured ribs may prevent participation in self-care.
Provide full bath and oral hygiene until patient's condition permits some participation.	Presence of rib fractures may make moving painful and anxiety provoking for patient initially so that care should be provided.
As condition improves, allow patient to bathe self using left side as able. Place bath basin, towels, soap, and personal hygiene articles	Bathing activities and doing own oral hygiene are tiring and require assistance to conserve energy. Bathing only easily reached body

Nursing Interventions	Rationales
in easy reach; wring and rinse cloth as needed; wash legs and back for patient.	areas by the patient prevents additional injury. Bathing the legs and back and other areas, as needed, permits checking skin integrity as well as prevents pain from stretching of fractured ribs to reach distant areas.
Assist with moving right arm and forearm.	There may be much edema, tenderness, pain, and drainage during first 3–5 postoperative days. Moving the arm aids recovery and hastens resolution of inflammation.
Encourage active exercises of both arms as healing progresses.	Exercises help maintain or regain muscle functions and provide positive evidence of progress toward recovery.
When condition permits, assist patient to be up and ambulate with right upper extremity in a sling.	Being up and ambulating stimulates systemic circulation to aid healing and should lead to discharge to home.
Teach steps of neurovascular checks to family and significant others (see Table 1.4, page 21).	Neurovascular checks may be required for a period after discharge to home.
Teach care of cast or wound as applicable.	Patient may only have closed reduction of the fractured humerus if it is reducible and able to hold reduction in a cast. If the fracture is a displaced, angulated fracture, it may not hold after reduction and most commonly will require an open reduction.

▶ NURSING DIAGNOSIS: *High Risk for Peripheral Neurovascular Dysfunction, Such as Compartment Syndrome*

Risk Factors

- Angulated, displaced fracture of the humerus (long bone)
- Chemical changes in blood serum

- Release of fat molecules into blood stream
- Fascial covering over muscle bundles

Patient Outcomes

The patient will

- not experience fat embolism syndrome.
- have no abnormal neurovascular changes or elevated compartment pressures in affected extremity.
- not require fasciotomy or cast removal.

Nursing Interventions	Rationales
Assess all parts of neurovascular checks—color, temperature, edema, pain, motor and sensory functions, capillary refill, and peripheral pulses—and compare with opposite arm.	Data from neurovascular checks provide evidence of status of inner tissues over time. See Table 1.4, page 21.
Carefully evaluate patient's complaints of pain: is pain in excess of expected; is it relieved with analgesics; is pain increased with passive stretch?	One sign of developing compartment syndrome is pain beyond expected amounts according to severity of injury and pain increased on passive stretch of distal tissues.
Elevate arm on pillow.	Elevation increases venous return and increases arterial inflow.
Apply ice packs or use cold pack to affected arm.	Ice decreases bleeding and causes vasoconstriction, lessening pain and bleeding into tissues.
Notify physician if injured area becomes markedly edematous.	A marked increase in edema may be indicative of venous obstruction, continued bleeding into tissues, or a developing compartment syndrome.
Measure compartment pressures per needle or catheter according to manufacturer's recommendations; notify physician of pressure readings.	Readings of compartment pressures vary according to technique used; however, pressure readings above 25–30 mm (or below patient's diastolic pressure, up to 50–60 mm Hg) signify developing compartment syndrome. Elevated pressures must be relieved in 4–6h

Nursing Interventions	Rationales
	to prevent muscle ischemia and muscle damage. The most common treatment is fasciotomy.
Prepare patient for surgical release of fascia if pressures continue to rise.	Increased venous pressures prevent arterial inflow leading to muscle death. The fascia hold the enclosed muscle tightly and must be cut to allow the muscle to expand and arterial inflow to be restored. The muscle belly is covered with sterile wet compresses after fasciotomy to prevent drying and infection from developing.
Explain care to patient/family both pre- and postoperatively.	Compartment syndrome is a severe complication and may result in loss of some muscle mass. The fascia is usually not closed again after the muscle swelling decreases, but the exposed muscle is usually covered with split-thickness skin grafts. Rehabilitation exercises must be done to restore muscle functions after the grafts have "taken" and the areas are healed.

DISCHARGE PLANNING/CONTINUITY OF CARE

- Arrange for follow-up physician's visit.
- Provide written guides for neurovascular checks.
- Review medications and side effects; provide written instructions for medication regimen.
- Refer to home health agency for nursing follow-up on fracture healing, rehabilitation exercises, and assistance with activities of daily living (ADL), if needed.

Clinical Clip

Gunshot wounds have become a major cause of musculoskeletal trauma because of the increase in violent crimes. The severity of gunshot wounds is determined by the velocity, trajectory, mass of the bullet, and firing distance. The velocity of a bullet determines the extent of cavitation and tissue deformation. High-velocity bullets cause a cavity around the bullet and bullet tract, which can be as much as 30–40 times the diameter of the bullet. If the bullet strikes a bone, bone fragments can become secondary missiles, crushing tissue and increasing the severity of the wound (Gross, Day, & Petrec, 1991).

Table 1.1 • Definitions, Causes, and Common Treatments for Minor Injuries

Name	Definition	Causes	Common Treatments
Contusion	A bruise with bleeding into the tissues; a black-and-blue area from disruption of capillaries	A bump, blow, or fall	Application of ice to site
Strain	Excessive stretch of a muscle, ligament, or tendon resulting in pain, soreness, and inability to use normally; may have first-, second-, or third-degree strain	Excessive use, pull, or stretch of tissue affected; may be from acute (sudden) or chronic use or overuse	Application of ice to area; temporary rest to part; use of mild analgesics
Sprain	Partial or complete tearing of fibers of a tendon or ligament in or around a joint; may have first-, second-, or third-degree sprain	Twist, fall, or overstretch of involved tissue	Application of ice; rest to part; use of cane or crutches; application of compression bandage; gradual increase in exercise and use of part. Third-degree tears require surgical restoration of continuity of affected tissues, followed by rehabilitative exercises.

Table 1.1 • *continued*

Name	Definition	Causes	Common Treatments
Subluxation	Partial dislocation of a bone from a joint	Direct or sideways force on bone or joint	Manual traction, to replace bone in joint; compression; immobilization with a splint; application of ice
Dislocation	Complete separation of the bones in a joint	Pressure severe enough to push or force a bone from a joint	Same as for subluxation, along with use of a sling for shoulder or elbow, or traction after a hip reduction

Table 1.2 • Descriptions of Types and Causes of Fractures

Type of Fracture	Descriptive Factors	Force or Energy Causing Fracture and Injury
Closed	Skin is closed but bone is fractured	Minor energy
Open	Skin is open, bone is fractured, and there may be trauma to soft tissues	Moderate to severe energy that is continuous and exceeds tissue tolerances
Greenstick	Break in only one cortex of the bone	Minor direct or indirect energy
Transverse	Horizontal break through the bone	Direct or indirect energy toward the bone
Spiral	Fracture curves around both cortices and may become displaced by twist	Direct or indirect twisting energy or force with the distal part held or unable to move
Oblique	Fracture at an oblique angle across both cortices	Direct or indirect energy with angulation and some compression
Comminuted	Fracture with more than two pieces; may have much associated soft tissue trauma	Direct crushing energy or force to tissue and bone

Table 1.2 • *continued*

Type of Fracture	Descriptive Factors	Force or Energy Causing Fracture and Injury
Compression	Fracture of bone which is squeezed or wedged together at one side	Compressive, axial energy or force applied directly from above the fracture site
Avulsed	Fracture that pulls bone and other tissue from their usual attachments	Direct energy or force with resisted extension of the bone and joint
Stress	Crack in one cortex of a bone	Repetitive direct energy or force as from jogging, running, or striking a lever or from osteoporosis
Pathologic	Transverse, oblique, or spiral fracture of a bone weakened by tumor presence	Minor energy or force, which may be direct or indirect
Linear	As a line so can be transverse or oblique	Minor or moderate energy or force directly to bone
Impacted	Fracture with one end wedged into the opposite or inside of the fractured fragment	Compressive, axial energy or force directly to the distal fragment

Source: From The Nursing Process in the Care of Adults with Orthopaedic Conditions, *3rd ed., by Mourad, L. A. and Droste, M. M., 1993, Albany, NY: Delmar. Copyright 1993 by Delmar Publisher Inc. Reprinted by permission.*

Table 1.3 • Stages and Characteristics of Fracture Healing

Stage	Characteristics
Hematoma formation/ inflammatory stage	Release of histamine, bradykinins, and serotonin into injury site with bleeding, causing a hematoma to form; thrombocytes and fibroblasts form a fibrin clot in 24–48h, slowing bleeding or causing it to stop; growth factors from platelets, macrophages, lymphocytes, and hematopoietic cells begin to form new blood vessels in the injured area; period lasts 7–21 days
Consolidation/ cartilagogenesis stage	Bone-forming cells, primarily osteoblasts, move into the fibrin meshwork to make new *bone*, not scar tissue, a phenomenon unique to bone and liver; no other tissues regenerate as themselves but form scar tissue;

Table 1.3 • *continued*

Stage	Characteristics
	osteoblasts intertwine with collagen connective tissue cells to form bone, to bridge the gap between the ends of the fractured bone; capillaries grow into blood vessels to bring nutrients and calcium into the area to strengthen the cartilage matrix into bone; period lasts up to 6 weeks or longer
Callus formation stage	This is a very vital period for fracture healing during which sufficient nutrients—oxygen, alkaline phosphatase, vitamins, carbohydrates, proteins, minerals, especially calcium, water, and growth factors such as insulin, a potent growth factor—must all be present in quantities to promote full healing; alkaline phosphatase is a key enzyme in the mineralization process; along with all of the above nutrients and growth factors, another critical element is the "right" amount of compression of the fracture fragments for healing to be complete; too little compression may lead to false bone formation, whereas too much compression may lessen oxygen supply and tension, resulting in bone-end absorption and creating too large a gap for the collagen/cartilage/bone fibers to bridge; bone cells which resorb bone cells, called osteoclasts, increase resorption where compressive forces are large; period of callus formation lasts 6 months or longer, depending on the type, site, and nutrient conditions given above
Remodeling stage	During this period, excess callus, if present, is absorbed, and the healing bone is reshaped along the lines of stress according to Wolff's law; new trabeculae are formed along these lines of stress, and the bone will become thicker and stronger according to its function; remodeling may continue up to 2 years after long bones are fractured

Table 1.4 • Parameters and Significance of Neurovascular Checks

Parameter	Significance
Color of affected and surrounding tissues	Indicates adequacy of circulation; color should be pinkish, not pale or white; injured tissues are usually paler than the contralateral tissues
Temperature of affected tissue	Indicates circulatory adequacy or perfusion; injured tissues are usually cooler than contralateral tissues
Capillary refill of nails	Refill in 2–4 s indicates normal capillary perfusion; initially, injured tissues may have normal refill, but gradual slowing may be noted with careful assessment; slowing to 4–6 s should be reported
Edema	Presence indicates venous stasis; injured tissues usually are noticeably more swollen than contralateral tissues
Range of motion or movement of tissues	Indicates amount or degree of limitation(s) of movement; injured tissues usually have decreased mobility (patient may hold the part to lessen pain)
Sensory functions (may not be diagnostic in newborn or very young baby)	Indicates pressure on nerves, noted by complaints of numbness, tingling, or "pins and needles" sensation
Complaints of pain	Indicates injury, pressure, or trauma to tissues; injured tissues usually are more painful than contralateral tissues
Peripheral pulses	Presence indicates arterial perfusion; absence of one or more peripheral pulses indicative of lack of arterial inflow
Affected and unaffected tissues bilaterally	Indicates specific tissue involved when compared with other side

Source: From Orthopedic Disorders *by L. Mourad, 1991, St. Louis, MO: Mosby-Yearbook. Copyright 1991 by C. V. Mosby. Reprinted by permission.*

Table 1.5 • Traction: Types, Principles and Purposes, and Considerations for Care

Type	Patient's Age	Amount of Weight	Purposes and Principles	Considerations for Care
Buck's extension (one or both legs)	Any Age; most commonly used in adults	5–8 lb/leg	Applied preoperatively for hip fractures; for "pulling"contracted muscles; for relieving muscle spasms of legs or back; patient usually lies in recumbent position; may be turned to either side if no fracture is present; if there is a fracture, patient is turned to unaffected side; pillows to back and between legs	Skin of older patients is more "friable" and subject to loosening because of less subcutaneous fat; patient's complaints of burning under tape, moleskin, or traction boot should be assessed; traction may be removed for skin care even in presence of fracture
Russell's (one or both legs)	Children 5 years or older to older adults	2–5 lb/leg	Applied for "pulling" contracted muscles; preoperatively for hip fractures; uses principle that "for every force in one direction, there is a an equal force in the opposite direction" for the pulley placement and amount of weight used, because weight pull is doubled	Patient is positioned on back for most effective pull; knee sling can be loosened for skin care and checking pulses in popliteal area
Pelvic belt or girdle (abdomen and pelvis are enclosed)	Adults or older adolescents	20–35 lb	Relieve muscle spasms and pain associated with "disc" conditions; pull is from iliac crests to relieve spasms	Patient may be positioned in Williams position, which permits 45° of flexion of the knees and hips to relax lumbosacral muscles; orders usually state to be "in traction 2h, out 2h" and out of traction at night; traction straps should not put pressure over sciatic nerves

Pelvic sling (under pelvis and buttocks like a hammock)	Adults	20–35 lb	For holding fractured pelvic bones; buttocks must be slightly off bed	Patients are very comfortable in the sling even with extensive pelvic bruising; they may become quite dependent on being in the sling, and gradual "weaning" may be required; the sling should be kept clean and dry, and the patient can be removed from the sling for care and toileting, if institutional policies permit
Cervical head halter (under chin, around face, and back of head)	Adults	5–15 lb	For relieving muscle spasms caused by degenerative or arthritic conditions in or of the cervical vertebrae; halter should be applied so pull comes from occipital area, not through chin portion	Patients may be in low or high Fowler's position depending on the purpose of the traction; halter is usually incorrectly positioned if the patient complains of pain of chin, teeth, or temporomandibular joint; the side straps usually should be adjusted to relieve these complaints; patients should be removed from the traction for sleeping; patients may also use this type of traction at home for cervical arthritic conditions

Table 1.5 • *continued*

Type	Patient's Age	Amount of Weight	Purposes and Principles	Considerations for Care
Cotrel's (cervical head halter and pelvic belt to pelvis)	Adolescents	5–7 lb to head halter and 10–20 lb to pelvic belt	For stretching muscles preoperatively for scoliosis; principle is to pull muscles and joints apart	Patient is put in this traction to relax muscles and curvature; should be in traction except for sleeping; rarely, patient may be placed in Cotrel's postoperatively, too, although less frequently because of newer operative techniques such as Harrington or Luque rod insertion
Dunlop's (lower humerus and forearm)	Children to adults	5–7 lb to humerus; 3–5 lb to forearm	For realigning fractures of the humerus; body is used for countertraction by slightly elevating side of bed of arm in traction; forearm is merely held at right angles to the humerus for comfort, by using Buck's extension to the forearm	Dunlop's can be totally skin traction by Buck's extension to the humerus or can be skeletal with a Steinmann pin inserted through the distal humerus; use of either depends on the patient's injury; traction to the *forearm* should be removed daily for skin care, pulse checks, and ROM exercises, since the forearm traction is merely a means to keep the forearm vertically at a right angle to the humerus; patients must have assistance during ADL because they are held flat on their backs; they can turn enough for back care only

Cervical via skull tongs (skull bones bilaterally)	Any age (most commonly young adults)	20–30 lb (depends on weight of patient)	To realign fractures of cervical vertebrae and to relieve pressure on cervical nerves; patient must be on a special bed or frame such as a CircOlectric bed or Stryker frame to facilitate care; traction weights must never be "lifted"; traction must be continuous	Patients with this traction may be severely injured, having either upper or lower spinal cord injury or complete transection, making them quadriplegics or paraplegics; neurovascular checks are required hourly to assess progression or relief of symptoms; patients also may develop paralytic ileus (therefore are given nothing by mouth), may have a nasogastric tube inserted to suction, and have an indwelling urinary catheter; pin care is done every 4 h: soak sterile applicators in a half-strength solution of hydrogen peroxide and normal saline; apply to each pin site; allow to stand 5–10 min; use soaked applicators to remove drainage; dry sites; apply antibiotic or antiseptic ointment to pin sites if ordered

Table 1.5 • *continued*

Type	Patient's Age	Amount of Weight	Purposes and Principles	Considerations for Care
Balanced suspension to femur (Steinmann pin or Kirschner wire inserted through upper tibia; thigh and leg are suspended in a splint and leg attachment)	Any age from 3 years	20–35 lb	For realignment of fractures of the femur; to overcome muscle spasms associated with fractures of the femur; suspension of the thigh and leg is "balanced" by countertraction attached to the top of the thigh splint with weights equal to those of suspension (usually 7–8 lb)	Patients in this traction should be recumbent for best effects; they can turn approximately 30° to either side briefly for back care or can lift themselves using the trapeze and by using the uninjured leg and foot; neurovascular checks are vital to assess circulatory status and to prevent compartment syndrome

Source: From Clinical nursing *by Thompson, J. M., McFarland, G. K., Hirsch, J. E. & Tucker, S. M., St. Louis, MO: Mosby-Yearbook. Copyright 1993 by C. V. Mosby. Reprinted by permission.*

Table 1.6 • Principles of Care of a Person in an External Fixator

Prior to application of the fixator

- If patient's condition permits, show the parts of the type of fixator to be applied or show a picture of the fixator to the patient and family

Prepare the patient physically and psychologically

- Do preoperative care if fixator is to be applied in the surgical site
- Clarify any concerns or questions from patient or family or refer them to physician as needed
- Explain upcoming events and time periods involved to lessen anxiety or concerns

After application of fixator and return to hospital room

- Assist with proper positioning of the patient and area in fixator; use pillows for support or elevation as needed
- Do neurovascular checks of area involved
- Check entrance/exit sites of transfixing pins for presence of the amount of drainage; initial drainage may be serosanguineous; small dressings may cover pin sites
- If fixator applied after open reduction of fractured bone, do usual postoperative care such as vital signs, intravenous therapy, antibiotic administration, intake and output, and other care as needed
- If prescribed, do pin site care, which varies per institution when patient is to be discharged
- Teach patient and family care of pin sites as prescribed by physician; care may be only checking each pin site for evidence of inflammation (redness, edema, clear drainage, or pain) and keeping areas clean and dry; if some drainage persists, some physicians suggest cleaning pin sites with applicators soaked in half-strength hydrogen peroxide/saline to loosen secretions, removing secretions, and drying with dry applicators; sites may then be covered with sterile dressings held in place with stretchy gauze (Kerlex); some physicians just want the pin sites covered with Kerlex gauze and changed every third day; put instructions in writing
- Secure prescription for analgesics for patient's pain; discuss effects and side effects
- Provide hospital nursing unit phone number for patient to call if questions arise
- Arrange for patient's next physician's visit; provide appointment card

REFERENCES

Behrman, S., Fabian, T., & Kudok, K. (1990). Improved outcome with femur fractures. Early vs. delayed fixation. *Journal of Trauma, 30,* 792.

Belinsky, J. D. (1993). Acetabular fracture: ORIF. *Orthopaedic Nursing, 12*(1), 42–50.

Grana, M. A., & Hines, R. (1992). Arthroscopic-assisted semitendinosus reconstruction of the anterior cruciate ligament. *American Journal of Knee Surgery, 5*(1), 16–22.

Gross, R.P., Day, T., & Petrec, C. (1991). Initial assessment and management of a patient with a gunshot wound to the femur. *Orthopaedic Nursing, 10*(6), 9–13.

Herzog, R. J. (1992). Imaging of the knee. *Orthopaedic Review, 21*(12), 1409–1417.

Keenan, M. A. E. (moderator), Botte, M. Jr., Hsu, J., Liebenberg, R., & Moore, T. J. (1993). Symposium: Orthopaedic management of patients with traumatic brain injuries. *Contemporary Orthopaedics, 27*(4), 357–398.

Maher, A. B., Salmond, S. W., & Pellino, T. (1993). *Orthopaedic nursing.* Philadelphia: Saunders.

Miller, M. D., Johnson, D. L., Harner, C. D., & Fu, F. H. (1993). Posterior cruciate ligament injuries. *Orthopaedic Review, 22*(11), 1201–1209.

Mourad, L. A. (1991). *Orthopedic disorders.* St. Louis: Mosby-Yearbook.

Mourad, L. A., & Droste, M.M. (1993). *The nursing process in the care of adults with orthopaedic conditions* (3rd ed.). Albany: Delmar.

O'Meara, P. M. (1992). Management of open fractures. *Orthopaedic Review, 21*(10), 1177–1185.

Perloff, J. J., McDermott, M. T., Perloff, K. G., Blue, P. W., Enzenhauer, R., Sieck, E., Chantelois, A. E., Dolbow, A., & Kidd, G. S. (1991). Reduced bone-mineral content is a risk factor for hip fractures. *Orthopaedic Review, 20*(8), 689–698.

Shea, K. P. (1992). Beware the "simple" rotator cuff tear. *Complications in Orthopedics, 8*(1), 297–303.

Shelbourne, K. D., & Porter, D. A. (1992) ACL-MCL injury: Non-operative management of the MCL tears with ACL reconstruction. *American Journal of Sports Medicine, 20*(2), 283–286.

Thompson, J. M., McFarland, G. K., Hirsch, J. E., & Tucker, S. M. (1993). *Clinical nursing.* St. Louis, MO: Mosby-Yearbook.

Williams, R. P., Friis, E. A., Cooke, F. W., McQueen, D. A., & Toohey, J. S. (1992). External fixation of unstable Malgaigne fractures: The comparative mechanical performance of a new configuration. *Orthopaedic Review, 21*(12), 1423–1430.

CASTS

A cast is a means of immobilizing a fractured bone or bones during the time needed for healing. The majority of casts are applied using gypsum or plaster-of-paris, but some may be made of fiberglass or cast tape.

Materials needed for application of a cast are usually on shelves in the cast application area or on portable carts for ease in accessibility and use.

ETIOLOGIES

- Disruption of ligament(s) with strain or sprain
- Fracture of one or more bones, with or without displacement

CLINICAL MANIFESTATIONS

- Break in one or more bones
- Injury to ligament resulting in hemorrhage in area or tear of fibers

CLINICAL/DIAGNOSTIC FINDINGS

- History of injury through accident, fall, or other cause
- Physical examination reveals loss of function of affected part, loss of normal anatomy, bruising, pain, and swelling at site
- Roentgenograms reveal disruption of normal bone anatomy, possible displacement of one or more bones

► NURSING DIAGNOSIS: *Impaired Physical Mobility*

Related To presence of fracture of one or more bones and cast

Defining Characteristics

- Complaint of acute pain
- Inability to use affected part or parts
- Presence of damp plaster cast or of fiberglass cast

Patient Outcomes

The patient will

- regain an intact bone or bones following healing.
- retain or maintain the cast without breaks or wetness.
- regain mobility of affected bone(s) with use of sling or ambulatory aid.
- retain as much muscle strength and mass as possible.

Nursing Interventions	Rationales
Place damp cast on soft but firm pillows to elevate cast and injured tissues.	Pillows should be firm to prevent deforming of cast. Elevation decreases bleeding and edema.
Apply ice bags or cold therapy to injured area.	Ice causes vasoconstriction to lessen bleeding.
Use palms of hands, not fingertips, to handle damp cast.	Fingertips can cause indentations in a damp cast which could cause pressure areas inside cast.
Keep a damp cast uncovered.	Covering a damp cast delays or prevents drying.
Assess range of motion (ROM) of muscles and joints.	Data indicate condition of tissues for planning care.
Mark any drainage that appears on cast.	Presence of drainage may signify infection, as this was a closed reduction. There should be no bleeding on outside of skin.
Teach and encourage patient to do muscle-setting exercises.	Muscle-setting exercises maintain and strengthen muscles and enhance circulation.
As needed, assist patient with ROM exercise to unaffected joints.	Range-of-motion exercises maintain healthy cartilage and other joint tissues.
Assist the patient to be up and ambulatory, as permitted. Apply a sling for a cast on an upper extremity, and assist with the use of a walker or crutches, as needed.	Being up and ambulating helps maintain muscle mass and strength.
Encourage intake of high-vitamin, high-protein, high-carbohydrate diet and 3,000 mL of fluid intake daily.	Persons with decreased mobility lose muscle mass unless proper nutrients are ingested. Vitamins A, C, and D are needed for bone

Nursing Interventions	Rationales
	healing and cellular growth. Proteins aid tissue and collagen growth and carbohydrates spare proteins for tissue buildup. Fluid intake is vital for all cell functions.

▶ NURSING DIAGNOSIS: *Acute Pain*

Related To new fracture and soft tissue injury

Defining Characteristics

- Angulated, displaced fracture of humerus or tibia
- Marked bruising and ecchymosis at fracture site

Patient Outcomes

The patient will

- experience pain controllable with medications.
- regain pain-free state over time and healing.

Nursing Interventions	Rationales
Assess for patient's complaints of pain: type, site, characteristics, duration, and intensity. Use pain scales (0–10 or 0–5) to help assess patient's pain.	Determining the particulars of the patient's pain helps to provide individualized care.
Reposition the patient, as needed.	Repositioning eases sore, painful muscles and joints.
Reapply warm (if 72 h or more after injury) or cold packs to site.	Cold lessens pressure on nerve endings to relieve pain.
Administer prescribed analgesic medications, initially around the clock.	Analgesics relieve acute pain. Around-the-clock administration helps maintain therapeutic blood levels.
Massage back several times daily.	Massage aids circulation and helps remove wastes from tired, aching muscles and tissues.

Nursing Interventions	Rationales
Explain the gradual decrease in painful episodes as healing progresses and inflammation is resolved.	Restoration of an intact bone through healing and clearing of inflammatory changes should remove painful stimuli.
Administer nonnarcotic, anti-inflammatory medications between dosages of narcotics.	Nonnarcotic, anti-inflammatory medications, such as ibuprofen or aspirin, hasten resolution of inflammation.

▶ NURSING DIAGNOSIS: *Self Care Deficit, Bathing/Hygiene*

Related To cast on upper extremity

Defining Characteristics

- Fracture of humerus
- Presence of cast on dominant arm

Patient Outcomes

The patient will

- be able to participate in self-care with assistance.
- regain independence following fracture healing, removal of cast, and rehabilitation exercises.

Nursing Interventions	Rationales
Assess patient's ability to use nondominant arm to participate in own care.	Patient may be able to do some parts of care with assistance using nondominant hand.
Arrange personal items for easy access; rinse and soap wash cloth for patient's use.	Assistance lessens patient's energy expenditure through needing to use nondominant side unaccustomedly.
Assist the patient with oral hygiene as needed.	Thorough oral hygiene aids intake of food and fluids and lessens possibility of oral infection.
When conditions permit, assist patient to shower or bath, covering cast in plastic bag.	Plaster casts must be kept dry to prevent weakening. Covering with a plastic bag keeps the cast dry.
Encourage patient to use own clothing, gowns, or shirts as able.	Use of personal items is helpful for the patient's well being.

▶ NURSING DIAGNOSIS: *High Risk for Impaired Skin Integrity*

Risk Factors
- Displaced fracture of humerus
- Long arm cast on upper extremity (arm and forearm)

Patient Outcomes
The patient will
- retain intact skin surfaces with no pressure areas.
- regain usual skin integrity after removal of cast.

Nursing Interventions	Rationales
Assess skin areas above and below cast ends for color, odor, temperature, pressure signs, edema, or changes in motor or sensory functions.	These signs give evidence of pressure on skin surfaces.
Encourage patient to exercise wrist and fingers.	Exercises help maintain circulation and strength in skin and subcutaneous tissues.
Listen to patient's complaints of feeling of tightness and pressure around elbow area in cast.	Tightness and pressure around elbow signify edema and could lead to development of pressure areas or other complications such as compartment syndrome.
Apply ice to elbow area of cast.	Ice causes vasoconstriction which lessens edema and thus should lessen tightness and pressure of tissues in cast.
Elevate cast with forearm higher than arm and shoulder.	Elevation increases venous return to lessen edema formation, thus lessening pressure and tightness.
Do all neurovascular checks q1h (see page 21 for checks and rationale for checks).	Data from checks indicate effects of ice and elevation.
Bathe areas above and below cast daily.	Bathing helps maintain clean, intact skin surfaces.
Assist patient to change positions q2–3h.	Position changes or weight shifts increase circulation and help maintain intact skin surfaces in all body areas.

Nursing Interventions	Rationales
Assist patient to be up with arm/cast in sling.	Ambulation aids circulation and helps maintain muscle mass, muscle strength, and skin integrity in the body. Use of a sling helps maintain proper position of the cast and fractured bone.
Observe patient for any diaphoresis or moisture on skin.	Diaphoresis would be present inside a cast if noted in other body areas. Such wetness could cause skin maceration and could lead to skin breakdown.
Monitor nutritional intake and fluid intake and output.	Daily nutritional and fluid intakes must be adequate for cell healing, bone regeneration and growth, and proper hydration and circulation to and from all cells, especially musculoskeletal and skin tissues.

▶ NURSING DIAGNOSIS: *High Risk for Additional Injury*

Risk Factors

- Unhealed fractured bone
- Wet, damp plaster cast

Patient Outcomes

The patient will

- experience no additional injury during period of cast.
- have complete healing of fracture.

Nursing Interventions	Rationales
Assess size and shape of cast and position of tissues in cast.	Assessment data help determine positioning or handling techniques.
Assess tissues above and below cast for evidence of rough cast edges, lacerations, or cuts.	Rough edges can cause cuts or lacerations in contiguous skin tissues, especially during application or prior to finishing edges of cast.

Nursing Interventions	Rationales
Gently elevate encased tissues on soft, firm pillows to heart level.	Elevation prevents additional edema formation and aids venous return.
Handle casted tissues under joints above and below injury site.	Supporting under these two joints prevents unsafe pressure on a wet cast and "levering" action of unstable bone on soft tissues or joint.
Keep cast uncovered until cast sounds hollow when thumped. Use a fan to aid drying of a large cast.	A damp cast sounds dull, whereas a dry cast sounds hollow when thumped. A fan aids drying by increasing air movement but should not be used if the patient has wounds or an incision under the cast, as microorganisms could be blown under the cast.
Keep the room temperature at 72–76 F (22–24 C) while cast is damp.	Having a damp cast, if large, may lower patient's body temperature and make him or her feel cold.
Reposition patient and cast q3–4h.	Repositioning aids drying of all parts of cast plus aids patient's circulation and prevents pressure areas.
Perform all neurovascular checks q1–2h for 24–48 h.	Neurovascular checks provide evidence of circulatory adequacy or of a developing complication such as compartment syndrome (see page 299 for discussion of compartment syndrome, and for neurovascular checks (see Table 1.4, page 21)).
Apply ice or cold therapy to site of injury under cast.	Ice lessens bleeding, lessens pain, and decreases edema formation.
Provide written home care instructions if patient is to be discharged.	Written instructions lessen the possibility of errors or omissions and provide for security and safety.
Discuss skin care after removal of cast; put instructions in writing (see Table 2.1, page 37).	After a period, usually 5–6 weeks if an adult, in a cast, the skin surfaces, muscles, and joints require special care to prevent excoriation or injury.

DISCHARGE PLANNING/CONTINUITY OF CARE

- Give the patient written instructions for wound, skin, or cast care, ROM exercises, and dietary intake.
- Make appointments for return to physician.
- Refer to community health nurses and, depending on the severity and extent of injuries, physical and occupational therapists.
- Instruct to notify physician if there are marked increase in pain, break in cast, numbness in part in cast, or inability to move distal tissues in cast.

Clinical Clip

The acronym RICE is used when treating acute injuries:

R = *R*est, to affected part or whole person

I = *I*ce, for vasoconstriction and to lessen pain

C = *C*ompression, brought about by use of elasticized bandages or application of a cast

E = *E*levation, which increases venous return, thus lessening edema formation

Clinical Clip

Neurovascular checks involve the following parameters:

Peripheral pulses—are they palpable?

Skin color at site

Presence of edema at site

Temperature of skin in affected area

Amount of pain in area

Motor functions in area

Sensory functions in area

Capillary refill

Comparing with contralateral tissues

Table 2.1 • Instructions for Post-Cast Removal Care

- Apply the full-strength solution of cold-water wash with enzymes, such as Woolite and Delicare, to the skin areas that had been in a cast; allow it to remain on skin for 20 minutes; enzymes loosen dead cells and fatty and crusty debris without injuring underlying cells
- After 20 min, have the patient immerse the part in warm water, such as in a shower or bath, and gently rinse off the loosened debris, using a cloth, not fingernails; caution patient to rinse gently and not to rub or scrub surfaces
- Rinse the area well, then pat dry with a towel, being careful on the tender skin areas
- Have the patient apply a moisturizing skin lotion to the area
- Instruct the patient to repeat the cleansing steps in 24 h, if needed, after which the skin areas should be in their usual precast condition
- Explain that there may be some swelling or edema of the affected tissues and that the patient should elevate the part for the next 24–48 h; occasionally, wrapping the part with elastic bandages also eases swelling
- Explain that there might be some soreness, weakness, or tenderness in the muscles and joints that had been in the cast and reuse should be begun slowly; the patient may need to take a nonnarcotic analgesic (aspirin or acetaminophen) until the soreness is eased; generally, it takes twice as long to regain strength as the part had been in a cast

REFERENCES

Connolly, J. F. (1993). Avoiding pitfalls in forearm fracture management. *Journal of Musculoskeletal Medicine, 10*(1), 72–82.

Giordano, C. (1993). How do fracture blisters affect fracture care? *Orthopedics Today. 13*(1), 1, 12.

Merchan, E. C. R., Breton, A. F., Galindo, E., Peinado, J. F., & Beltran, J. (1992). Plaster cast versus Clyburn external fixation for fractures of the distal radius in patients under 45 years of age. *Orthopaedic Review, 21*(10), 1203.

Mourad, L. A., & Droste, M. M. (1993). *The nursing process in the care of adults with orthopaedic conditions* (3rd ed.). Albany: Delmar.

Rettig, A. C., Alexy, C., & Malone, K. (1992). Protective devices for hand and wrist injuries in athletes. *Journal of Musculoskeletal Medicine, 9*(12), 62–75.

Degenerative Joint Conditions

Degenerative joint conditions affect persons as they live and age. Degenerative conditions result from use of musculoskeletal tissues, trauma, developmental conditions, or wear and tear or other influences on muscles, bones, and joints and tend to become progressively more painful and incapacitating over time, with or without treatment.

Primarily, cartilage covering the ends of bones is the tissue involved in degenerative conditions. With cartilage deterioration, other joint tissues are secondarily affected leading to the condition referred to as degenerative joint disease.

Osteoarthritis is the major degenerative joint disease. It affects millions of older adults and is a major health condition, resulting in billions of health care expenditures.

OSTEOARTHRITIS

Osteoarthritis is a degenerative condition of the cartilage in a joint.

ETIOLOGIES

- Primary osteoarthritis: may be due to abnormal regeneration of cartilage due to a genetic deficit or excessive stress, or wear and tear on the joint cartilage
- Secondary osteoarthritis: may follow or result from trauma, infection, or congenital dysplasia in a joint, such as congenital hip dysplasia, fractures, and endocrine or metabolic disorders
- Obesity: may contribute to added stress on joint cartilage
- Aging: occurs more frequently in persons over age 50
- Sex: occurs slightly more frequently in women than men

CLINICAL MANIFESTATIONS

- Deformity of joint or joints; usually one joint may be more prominently affected than others
- Gait changes: may develop a lurching gait if hip or knee involved
- Limitation of joint movements
- Major weight-bearing joints such as hip or knee usually affected before joints of upper extremities
- Pain in or around a joint, dull or aching in type, may wake person from sleep and interfere with rest
- Presence of Heberden's nodes in distal joints of fingers or Bouchard's nodes in proximal interphalangeal joints
- Shortening of affected joint(s) or limb
- Stiffness and edema of affected joint

CLINICAL/DIAGNOSTIC FINDINGS

- Erythrocyte sedimentation rate normal (done to rule out systemic disease)
- Magnetic resonance imaging may show osteonecrosis of femoral head if hip joint affected

- Radiographs of affected joint(s) show decreased joint space, loss of joint cartilage, sclerotic bone, bone cysts, osteophytes, or bone spurs with or without lipping of bone
- Synovial fluid analysis: usually clear and colorless; no crystals; occasional white blood cells (up to 200 or more)

▶ NURSING DIAGNOSIS: *Impaired Physical Mobility*

Related To degenerative joint processes

Defining Characteristics

- Inability to use joint/affected tissues normally or without pain due to stiffness or deformity of joint
- Presence of limp and joint weakness due to loss of cartilage and normal bone structure; joint may give way

Patient Outcomes

The patient will

- regain joint movements with minimal limitations or pain.
- regain restful sleep patterns.
- be compliant with medication regimen without experiencing distressing side effects.

Nursing Interventions	Rationales
Assess amount of joint movements, presence of deformity, stiffness, edema, and pain; compare with contralateral joint.	External appearance may or may not be indicative of internal pathology in joint structures, but external appearances can be compared to usual normals for particular joint.
Observe patient's use of affected joint(s), use of ambulatory aid, and unwillingness to use affected joint(s).	Observation of patient's use and activities helps determine needs and limitations. Ambulatory aid lessens stress on joint during weight-bearing activities.
Assist patient to change positions; provide pillows to prop in comfortable positions.	Assistance eases stress on weakened joint(s); use of pillows lessens muscle effort to maintain comfortable positions.
Assist patient with activities of daily living (ADL) as needed.	Assistance lessens stress on weakened joints and tissues.

Nursing Interventions	Rationales
Teach proper use of cane or crutches as prescribed.	A cane is used in the hand opposite the affected limb to resemble normal walking as much as possible. Use of crutches requires learning proper "gait" techniques.

▶ NURSING DIAGNOSIS: *Acute Pain*

Related To degenerative or destructive processes in affected joints

Defining Characteristics

- Hesitates to use joint(s) through normal range of motion (ROM)
- Holds joint in position of comfort
- Limps when weight-bearing; uses arms and hands to assist self when rising to lessen stress on joint and possible pain
- Verbalizes discomfort and presence of dull, aching pain in or around affected joint(s); states pain wakes him or her

Patient Outcomes

The patient will

- experience relief of pain with medications without distressing side effects.
- regain restful sleep.
- regain limited ROM of affected joint(s) with medications and/or surgical procedures.

Nursing Interventions	Rationales
Assess site(s), amount, duration, and type of pain; assess efforts at pain relief and results.	Pain is an individual experience and its extent must be individually determined. Results of pain relief efforts help determine future strategies.
Administer prescribed medications q4h; note effects of medications.	Medications may be analgesics such as aspirin based or non-steroidal anti-inflammatory. Therapeutic blood levels are maintained by regular administration as required.

Nursing Interventions	**Rationales**
Assist to positions of comfort as needed; assist with ROM exercises as tolerated.	Repositioning eases strain on tired or weakened muscles and joints. ROM exercises help maintain muscle strength.
Apply heat, cold, or other treatments such as diathermy as prescribed.	Pain is often relieved with use of heat and cold applications by vasodilation or vasoconstriction (see Table 3.1, page 45).
Encourage weight loss if overweight.	Obesity increases stress on joints.
Teach patient side effects of prescribed medications.	Common side effects are listed in Table 3.2, page 47.
Discuss proposed surgical procedures as appropriate.	Proposed surgery may be total joint replacement, spinal fusion, or prosthetic insertion (see Chapters 19 and 29).
Discuss and teach about strategies for pain relief such as relaxation techniques, imagery, diversional activities.	Relaxation of muscles and diversion or distraction provide pain relief for varying periods.

▶ NURSING DIAGNOSIS: *Altered Role Performance*

Related To limitations of movements and pain

Defining Characteristics

- Inability to engage in regular family or social activities as desired
- Inability to maintain usual employment activities or functions

Patient Outcomes

The patient will

- regain usual family or social activities after treatment.
- return to usual employment roles and activities.

Nursing Interventions	Rationales
Assess effects of joint involvement and pain on usual roles.	Data are necessary for individualized care.
Determine usual roles in family and in social activities.	Data help determine effects of limitations and pain.
Assist patient to identify strengths and potential changes needed, if appropriate.	Realistic appraisals of strengths and/or needed changes are growth factors.
Encourage patient to express concerns or feelings regarding role expectations.	Expression of concerns or feelings helps in clarifying needs for role adaptation.
Teach problem-solving skills if appropriate.	Adjustments in role performance may be needed due to progressive nature of osteoarthritis.
Discuss long-term medical treatment plan.	Clarification of long-term care eases concerns or anxieties about upcoming events or quality of life.

DISCHARGE PLANNING/CONTINUITY OF CARE

- Refer to home health care personnel for follow-up assessment of ambulation, exercise regimen, and wound healing.
- Clarify prescribed medication regimen and review side effects of medications.
- Arrange for follow-up physician's visit.

Table 3.1 • Therapeutic Uses of Cold and Heat

Primary Effects of Cold	Purpose(s)	Type of Application
Vasoconstriction	Decrease circulation to decrease bleeding	Ice bag; hypothermia; iced irrigations
Decrease circulation	Decrease tissue metabolism and decrease edema formation	Ice bags; cool bath with wet cloths or towels; cold compresses
Decrease temperature	Slow metabolism or suppuration (decrease inflammation	Temperature sponge bath (alcohol in water); ice bags; hypothermia
Decrease pain	Anesthesia to area	Hypothermia; ice to lower sensitivity

Table 3.1 • *continued*

Primary Effects of Heat	Purpose(s)	Type of Application
Vasodilation	Increase circulation and improve tissue oxygenation; hasten removal of irritants and wastes	Hot-water bag or bottle; infrared lamp; heating pads
Muscle relaxation	Decrease muscle spasm	Whirlpool bath; diathermy
Relief of pain	Decrease edema and spasm, increase removal of wastes	Heating pads, hot packs, paraffin "baths"
Remove external debris, drainage, and necrotic tissues; hasten suppuration	Cleanse area; heal area by removal of inflammatory products, wastes, or localizing inflammation	Moist, warm compresses (wet to dry compresses); Hubbard tank bath; whirlpool; sitz bath
Provide heat or warmth locally and/or systemically	Warm body and tissues; assist drying as with casts	Hot-water bottle; heat cradle; heating pad

Source: From The nursing process in the care of adults with orthopaedic conditions, *3rd. ed., by Mourad, L.A. and Droste, M.M., 1993, Albany, NY: Delmar.*

Table 3.2 • Medications Commonly Used for Musculoskeletal Conditions

Name of Medications	Adult Dosage (Orally)	Side Effects/ Adverse Reactions	Conditions Used
		Salicylates	
Aspirin, plain or buffered	600–3,000 mg/d	Anorexia, nausea, vomiting, gastric distress, gastrointestinal bleeding, decrease in clotting, ringing in ears (tinnitus)	Arthritis, all types; sports injuries (sprains, tennis elbow)
Choline magnesium trisalicylate (Trilisate)	250–1,000 mg b.i.d. or t.i.d.	Anorexia, nausea, headache, gastric distress	Low back pain; arthritis, all types
Choline salicylate (Arthropan)	2,000–3,000 mg t.i.d.	Same as for choline magnesium trisalicylate	Arthritis, all types
Salsalate (Disalcid)	1,000–3,000 mg/d	Same as for choline magnesium trisalicylate	Arthritis, all types
		Nonsteroidal Anti-inflammatory Drugs	
Ibuprofen (Motrin)	400 mg q.i.d.	Anorexia, nausea, vomiting, gastric distress, gastrointestinal bleeding, headache, dizziness, edema, fluid retention, skin rash, diarrhea or constipation, blurred vision, anemia	Arthritis, all types; low back pain
Fenoprofen (Nalfon)	600–3,200 mg/d	Same as for ibuprofen plus dysuria, cystitis, hematuria, proteinuria	Rheumatoid arthritis
Naproxen (Naprosyn)	250–750 mg/d	Same as for ibuprofen plus dysuria, cystitis, hematuria, proteinuria	Rheumatoid arthritis

Table 3.2 • *continued*

Name of Medications	Adult Dosage (Orally)	Side Effects/ Adverse Reactions	Conditions Used
	Nonsteroidal Anti-inflammatory Drugs		
Sulindac (Clinoril)	150–400 mg/d	Same as for ibuprofen plus dysuria, cystitis, hematuria, proteinuria	Arthritis, all types; ankylosing spondylitis
Tolmetin (Tolectin)	400–2,000 mg/d	Same as for ibuprofen plus dysuria, cystitis, hematuria, proteinuria	Rheumatoid arthritis
Meclo-fenamate (Meclomen)	50–100 mg	Same as with ibuprofen	Arthritis, all types
Piroxicam (Feldene)	20 mg/d	Same as with ibuprofen, but peptic ulceration and bleeding can be severe	Arthritis, all types
Indomethacin (Indocin)	25–75 mg/d to 150–200 mg/d for some clients	Same as with ibuprofen	Arthritis, all types
Phenyl-butazone (Butazolidin)	300–400 mg/d	Same as with ibuprofen plus aplastic anemia	Rheumatoid arthritis
Oxyphen-butazone (Tandearil)	300–400 mg/d	Same as for phenylbutazone	Rheumatoid arthritis
Diflunisal (Dolobid)	500–1,000 mg/d	Same as with ibuprofen plus eyesight changes (patients should see an ophthalmologist frequently)	Osteoarthritis
Diclofenac (Voltaren)	25–75 mg, 2–4 times daily	Same as with ibuprofen	Rheumatoid arthritis; osteo-arthritis; ankylosing spondylitis

Table 3.2 • *continued*

Name of Medications	Adult Dosage (Orally)	Side Effects/ Adverse Reactions	Conditions Used
		Steroids	
Prednisone (Deltasone, Meticorten, Fernisone)	5–60 (or more) mg/d	Anemia; edema, hypertension; sodium retention; potassium excretion; alteration in carbohydrate, protein, and fat metabolism; osteoporosis; bruising; moon facies; cataracts; hirsutism	Rheumatoid arthritis
		Antigout	
Colchicine (Colsalide)	1–1.2 mg followed by 0.5–0.6 mg/h until pain is relieved or diarrhea occurs	Nausea, vomiting, diarrhea, abdominal cramping; with long-term administration: bone marrow depression, aplastic anemia	Acute attack of gout
Probenecid (Benemid)	250–500 mg/d	Headache, anorexia, nausea, vomiting, diarrhea, constipation, rash, fever	Gout, long-term therapy
Sulfinpyrazone (Anturane)	200–400 mg/d	As with probenecid	Gout, long-term therapy
Allopurinol (Zyloprim)	200–600 mg/d	Skin rash, fever, malaise, cataracts, nausea, vomiting, diarrhea, drowsiness	Gout, long-term therapy

Source: From The nursing process in the care of adults with orthopaedic conditions, *3rd. ed., by Mourad, L.A. and Droste, M.M., 1993, Albany, NY: Delmar. Copyright 1993 by Delmar Publishers Inc. Reprinted by permission.*

REFERENCES

Bluestone, R. (1993). Assessing the patient with osteoarthritis: A regional approach. *Journal of Musculoskeletal Medicine, 10*(12), 46–54.

Dowd, S. B. (1993). The radiographic appearance of gout. *Orthopaedic Nursing, 12*(1), 53–55.

Fudman, E. J., & Fox, I. H. (1993). When clinical clues point to gout. *Journal of Musculoskeletal Medicine, 10*(2), 64–76.

Greene, M. K., & Rochberg, M. C. (1993). The epidemiology of osteoarthritis: What are the risk factors? *Journal of Musculoskeletal Medicine, 10*(5), 30–37.

Hunder, G. G., Kaye, R. L., & Williams, R. C. (1993). Osteoarthritis, osteoporosis, fibromyalgia: Advances in understanding and management. *Journal of Musculoskeletal Medicine, 10*(9), 16–32.

Mourad, L. A., & Droste, M. M. (1993). *The nursing process in the care of adults with orthopaedic conditions* (3rd ed.). Albany: Delmar.

Nelson, B. W. (1993). A rational approach to the treatment of low back pain. *Journal of Musculoskeletal Medicine, 10*(5), 67–82.

Overgaard, S., & Solgaard, D. (1989). Osteoarthritis after Colles' fracture. *Orthopedics, 12*(3), 413–416.

Robb, W. J. III (1993a). Hip fracture disease: Coping with a contemporary epidemic. *Journal of Musculoskeletal Medicine, 10*(12), 12–24.

Robb, W. J. III (1993b). Preventing hip fracture: Seven steps you can take. *Journal of Musculoskeletal Medicine, 10*(12), 12–24.

Summers, M. N., Haley, W. E., & Reveille, J. D. (1988). Why the OA patient says it hurts when clinically it shouldn't—and vice versa. *Arthritis and Rheumatism, 31*(2), 204–209.

DEGENERATIVE DISC CONDITIONS

Conditions within the vertebrae may lead to degenerative disc conditions which contribute to low back pain and pain in other areas of the vertebral column or contiguous musculoskeletal tissues. Radiation of pain may also cause functional changes in distal tissues such as the hand or fingers, and foot or toes.

ETIOLOGIES

- Aging: occur more frequently over age 40
- Congenital anomalies, such as spondylolisthesis or scoliosis
- Employment: more common in persons who do heavy lifting, turning, reaching, standing, or sitting for long periods
- Infection, such as discitis or osteomyelitis
- Musculoskeletal laxity of paraspinal muscles or ligaments or abdominal muscles
- Obesity
- Osteoarthritis
- Osteoporosis
- Male gender more than female
- Trauma

CLINICAL MANIFESTATIONS

- Change in lordosis in lumbosacral area
- Deformity of vertebral column
- Diffuse back pain in specific area of neck or back that may or may not radiate to contiguous or distal parts
- Fever, low grade
- Listing or bending to one side
- Obesity: over recommended weight for height
- Point tenderness along paraspinal areas

- Postmenopausal female
- Protruding abdomen

CLINICAL/DIAGNOSTIC FINDINGS

- History of sudden neck or back pain with a sneeze, with sudden twist or turn, or when lifting an unexpectedly heavy article
- History of osteomyelitis
- Physical examination showing tightness and muscle spasms of cervical or lumbosacral muscles
- Pain, radiating down arm or leg
- Loss of normal reflexes
- Roentgenograms showing osteoarthritic changes in cervical, thoracic, or lumbosacral vertebrae
- Previously diagnosed osteoporosis
- Male sex: more common to have ruptured disc
- Computerized tomography (CT) or magnetic resonance imaging (MRI) showing ruptured disc with pressure on spinal nerve, decreased bone density, spondylolisthesis or scoliosis, or disc inflammation

▶ NURSING DIAGNOSIS: *Acute Pain*

Related To degeneration and rupture of nucleus pulposus

Defining Characteristics

- Muscle spasms with movements
- Pain, eased with bedrest
- Pain, sharp and constant in lumbosacral area (most commonly) or in cervical area of neck
- Point tenderness, at times
- Radiation of pain to shoulders, arms, hips, or down thighs to legs

Patient Outcomes

The patient will

- regain a pain-free state or have minimal pain controlled by nonnarcotic medications after treatments.
- retain major muscle functions during treatment period.
- experience relief of ruptured disc with treatments.

Nursing Interventions	Rationales
Assess site(s) of pain, its type, characteristics, duration, alleviation or exacerbation, and severity.	Pain related to an acute disc rupture is usually severe, is constantly present, tends to be referred to as "burning", is somewhat relieved by lying down with knees bent, and is exacerbated by trying to rise to a standing position, turning, or twisting. Pain of discitis is more diffuse and dull but constant in area of inflammation. Pain of osteoarthritis, osteoporosis, spondylolisthesis, or scoliosis tends to be dull, relieved by lying or sitting, and localized to lower back and hip areas. Ninety-five percent of ruptures of discs occur between L_5 and S_1, with the remaining 5% occurring in the cervical or other lumbar areas.
Assess motor, sensory, or reflex functions.	With a ruptured disc, motor changes are related to the muscles involved, with slight weakness noted. Muscle spasms are common with an acute, sudden ruptured disc. Sensory changes may include complaints of numbness, tingling, "pins and needles" along affected spinal nerve root, and pain along the sciatic and peroneal nerve pathways to thigh, calf and foot or down arm to fingers if cervical disc is ruptured. The reflexes are decreased or absent. Reflex changes are uncommon in discitis. Sensory deficits cause marked discomfort because of the persistent numbness or burning sensations.
Assist patient to maintain prescribed bed position; use pillows or knee gatch positions to assist maintaining position.	The prescribed position may be 45° elevation of the head of bed and 45° elevation of the knees or knee gatch, a position known as

Nursing Interventions	Rationales
	the Williams position. Pillows under the knees may be used instead of knee gatch elevation. Bedrest is also commonly prescribed following low back pain associated with a ruptured disc. Bedrest may vary from 3 to 5 days or longer.
Administer prescribed anti-inflammatory and nonnarcotic analgesics.	Anti-inflammatory medications (see Table 3.2, page 47) relieve pain by lessening inflammatory changes, and nonnarcotic analgesics reduce perceptions of pain. These medications may be alternated and are usually given q3–4h to maintain therapeutic blood levels.
Assist patient to participate in physical therapy program.	Physical therapy exercises, ultrasound, or other therapies are usually prescribed when acute pain is manageable or inflammation is lessened. These exercises and ultrasound also ease inflammation, thus also lessening pain.

NOTE: See page 283 for nursing diagnosis of chronic pain.

▶ NURSING DIAGNOSIS: *Impaired Physical Mobility*

Related To pressure of ruptured disc on spinal nerves, muscle spasms, "flat" back, bedrest, and pain as described above

Defining Characteristics

- Decreased or absent reflexes of affected tissues
- Inability to do activities of daily living (ADL) and work activities
- Inability to rise without using hands on thighs or on furniture or without another person
- Inability to walk without muscle spasms in neck or back
- Listing to one side
- Loss of normal lumbar lordosis causing "flat" back
- Presence of numbness or tingling in one or both thighs, legs, or feet

Patient Outcomes

The patient will

- regain usual mobility with treatments.
- regain some lumbar lordosis after relief of muscle spasms.
- regain some reflexes after relief of pressure on nerves.
- experience relief of numbness and tingling after treatments.
- return to ADL and employment.

Nursing Interventions	Rationales
Assess physical mobility: ability to rise to standing position, sit down, walk for selected distance, and position when walking, sitting, or standing; observe patient from front, side, and back when standing or walking.	Muscle spasms and pain greatly limit the patient's ability to rise, stand straight, walk, and sit down. Use of hands on thighs (called quadriceps gait) may be needed when rising or patient may use furniture or assistance from another person to rise, stand, or sit down.
Assist patient as needed to change positions; use pillows to back when on side and under knees when on back.	Placing pillows provides support to aid in maintaining a desired position. Pillows under knees lessen strain on weakened muscles and lessen muscle spasms.
Allow sufficient time for patient to move, turn, rise, or walk.	Hurrying a patient may cause frustration or anger. With sufficient time, the patient can maintain some independence.
Anticipate need for anti-inflammatory/muscle-relaxant medications as prescribed.	These medications are given around the clock to lessen inflammation and to relieve muscle spasms.
Apply pelvic belt traction, if prescribed.	Pelvic belt traction is used to provide some stretch to lower back muscles to reduce pain and spasms. Up to 25 or more pounds of weight may be applied (see page 22 for discussion of pelvic belt traction).
Secure consultation with physical therapists for appropriate exercises and other therapies as prescribed.	Consultation with specialists helps assure that optimal therapies will be used to aid patient's recovery.
Monitor effects of medications and other therapies on motor and	A combination of therapies appears most beneficial to hasten

Nursing Interventions	Rationales
sensory functions and relief of symptoms.	resolution of inflammation, when or if possible.
Prepare patient for surgical repair or disc ablation or removal, if surgical option chosen.	Various surgical therapies (see pages 257–285) are available if bedrest, medications, and other therapies do not relieve pressure on nerves or relieve pain.

▶ NURSING DIAGNOSIS: *Self-Care Deficit—Bathing/Hygiene/Grooming*

Related To bedrest, neck or low back pain, and muscle spasms

Defining Characteristics

- Limited ability to do ADL because of muscle spasms
- Limited ability to turn self from side to side
- Presence of numbness and tingling in neck, shoulder, arm, thigh, or leg

Patient Outcomes

The patient will

- participate in self-care as able.
- regain full self-care following treatments.

Nursing Interventions	Rationales
Assess patient's ability to participate in bathing and grooming.	Data provide basis for subsequent interventions.
Arrange bathing and hygiene equipment and supplies for ease in reaching or use; assist with use as needed if has limited use of one arm or if muscle spasms limit movements.	Patient may be able to do portions of self-care if equipment is readily available and partial assistance given.
Arrange oral hygiene supplies and assist as needed.	Patient's limitations require assistance for thorough care.
Assist patient to turn for back care and position changes.	Turning may precipitate muscle spasms causing reluctance to move. Repositioning lessens muscle tiredness and increases circulation to all body cells.

Nursing Interventions	Rationales
Supply comb and personal items as desired; encourage use of own pajamas or gowns.	Use of personal items to aid grooming gives patient a sense of well-being and individuality.

▶ NURSING DIAGNOSIS: *Altered Role Performance*

Related To degenerative disc condition in neck or lower back

Defining Characteristics

- Required bedrest
- Pelvic belt traction or cervical head halter traction
- Hospitalization for acute rupture of cervical or lumbar disc

Patient Outcomes

The patient will

- experience relief of symptoms after treatments.
- return to usual roles after treatments and rehabilitation.

Nursing Interventions	Rationales
Assess necessary alterations in roles because of ruptured disc in neck or back.	Data are useful for all health team members for planning individualized care.
Assess motor and sensory functions and alterations related to arm, shoulder, neck, low back, hips, leg, thigh, or foot.	A disc can rupture in four directions—laterally, posteriorly, anteriorly, or obliquely—causing symptoms depending on if or where nerve pressure is involved. Motor functions may be minor to major weakness. Sensory changes vary from minimal numbness to marked paresthesia, pins-and-needles complaints, or numbness.
Discuss usual roles and employment settings.	Because of ruptured disc, treatments, and rehabilitation, the patient may require a change in employment settings, equipment, or other modifications.

Nursing Interventions	Rationales
Assist the patient with application of head halter traction or pelvic belt traction as prescribed.	Bedrest and specific skin traction are two initial treatments for ruptured discs.
Administer prescribed anti-inflammatory and muscle-relaxant medications as prescribed.	Use of these medications is part of the treatment regimen to help rehabilitate the patient.
Seek consultation with physical therapists for active and passive exercise programs, ultrasound, massage or other therapies.	Medical treatments for ruptured discs are varied according to individual patient needs.
Assist with ambulation when allowed up.	Bedrest weakens or lessens muscle strength and the patient should be assisted for safety.
Confer with and coordinate efforts of health team members (social worker, orthotist, physical and occupational therapist, and dietitian) as necessary.	Specialized services should be utilized to help the patient regain health and return to usual roles after treatments.
If to be discharged without surgical intervention, provide patient with written instructions for medication administration, diet, traction, or exercises.	Written instructions help assure the patient will be able to follow proper/desired techniques and provide safety.
Complete a continuity-of-care referral prior to discharge.	Provides for continuity and security in follow-up care.

▶ NURSING DIAGNOSIS: *Knowledge Deficit*

Related To unexpected and suddenness of condition

Defining Characteristics

- Hospitalization in acute discomfort and pain
- Sudden, severe pain and muscle spasms in neck or lower back
- Unfamiliar terms such as osteoarthritis, bulging or herniated disc, ruptured nucleus pulposus, pelvic belt or head halter traction, ultrasound, back belt, neck collar, and muscle-relaxant or anti-inflammatory medications

Patient Outcomes

The patient will

- develop understanding of condition, its treatments, and possible outcomes after explanations and teaching.
- experience relief of anxiety after learning situations.

Nursing Interventions	Rationales
Assess patient's understandings after physician's explanations.	Patient may have some understanding of condition after initial explanations.
Listen to and clarify any questions from patient or family.	Patient may be hesitant to ask questions when in pain or shock of suddenness of condition. As anxiety lessens and initial shock is relieved, patient may ask more pertinent questions.
Use charts or diagrams when providing explanations.	Patients learn using a variety of resources.
Continue to clarify new or upcoming diagnostic procedures or treatments.	Patient's anxiety may increase with new or potentially painful exams or treatments. Knowing what to expect eases anxiety and helps assure patient's cooperation.
Teach patient how to apply head halter or pelvic belt traction, if prescribed.	Patient in either type of traction should know how to apply and remove it for safety and security reasons. Patients are usually "in 2 hours, out 2 hours, and out at night" (see page 22 for discussion of each type of traction).
Discuss home care and follow-up care, if to be discharged without surgical repair; complete continuity-of-care referral.	Home care may include exercises, physical therapy, medications, and rest. Continuity of care is vital for thorough care.
Schedule follow-up visit with physician.	Appointment helps assure follow-up care.

NOTE: Surgical care for a ruptured disc is given on pages 257–285.

DISCHARGE PLANNING/CONTINUITY OF CARE

- Refer to community health nurses for follow-up of compliance with prescribed medication and rest/exercise regimens
- Make referral for physical therapy for prescribed exercise program

REFERENCES

Anderson, L. (1989). Educational approaches to management of low back pain. *Orthopaedic Nursing, 8*(1), 43–46.

Chase, J. A. (1992). Outpatient management of low back pain. *Orthopaedic Nursing, 11*(1), 11–20.

Fischgrund, J. S., & Montgomery, D. M. (1993). Diagnosis and treatment of discogenic low back pain. *Orthopaedic Review,* 22(3), 311–318.

Salmond, S. W., Mooney, N. E., & Verdisco, L. A. (1991). *Core curriculum for orthopaedic nursing* (2nd ed.). Pitman, NJ: Janetti.

Inflammatory Conditions

Inflammatory conditions of musculoskeletal tissues account for marked morbidity in persons from early ages through older adult years. Many inflammatory diseases which involve these tissues are autoimmune in origin. Others have genetic causes. Inflammatory diseases also, at times, shorten lives through their multiple organ involvement and inflammatory effects.

RHEUMATOID ARTHRITIS

Rheumatoid arthritis (RA) is a systemic disease presently considered to be an autoimmune disease. It is noted by inflammation of the connective tissues of the body, such as the tissues in joints, heart, lungs, kidneys, and skin. There is a marked familial tendency in RA. It affects women 3 : 1 over men, primarily during the ages of 25 and 55 years. A juvenile RA is called Still disease.

This presentation will focus on the effects of RA on the tissues in and around the joints.

ETIOLOGIES

- Autoimmune origin, although research is focusing also on a genetic etiology for RA
- Estrogens (female hormones), which may play a role in the pathogenesis or expression of RA
- Genetic predisposition
- Presence of human leukocyte antigen (HLA) DRB1 genes, which can identify persons at risk for development of RA (D'Cruz & Hughes, 1993)
- Presence of HLA-DR4 marker, which has strong relation to RA

CLINICAL MANIFESTATIONS

Four of the following seven criteria must be present for the classification of RA (D'Cruz & Hughes, 1993):

- Arthritis of hand joints, at least one joint swollen
- Arthritis of three or more joint areas simultaneously
- Morning stiffness, lasting at least 1 h before lessening
- Rheumatoid nodules, subcutaneous nodules over bony prominences or extensor surfaces
- Serum rheumatoid factor shows abnormal amounts
- Symmetric arthritis of same joints on both sides of body

CLINICAL/DIAGNOSTIC FINDINGS

- Erythrocyte sedimentation rate above normal levels
- Hemoglobin decreased, indicative of anemia

- History of patterns of joint swelling and pain with morning stiffness and symmetric joint involvement; profound fatigue and muscle/joint weakness
- Joint deformities with limited extension
- Muscle wasting, consistent with severity of synovitis
- Positive serum rheumatoid factor (seen in about 95% of patients)
- Red blood cell count below normal levels
- Roentgenographic findings include erosions or bony decalcification localized to or most marked adjacent to involved joints
- Subcutaneous nodules, commonly at olecranon and proximal ulna, finger extensor surfaces, and Achilles tendon
- Synovial fluid analysis may show immune complexes and elevated white blood cell counts (WBCs)
- Synovial membrane biopsy may show pannus formation and inflammatory changes
- Tenosynovitis of extensor tendons and sheaths
- Weight loss
- WBC levels elevated over all cell types

▶ NURSING DIAGNOSIS: *Activity Intolerance*

Related To anemia, muscle weakness, and fatigue

Defining Characteristics

- Increased pulse and respiratory rates on exertion due to anemia
- Increasing lethargy and tiredness over 4–5 h daily
- Malaise
- Muscle/joint weakness
- Paleness

Patient Outcomes

The patient will

- attain satisfactory (11.5–12 g) levels of hemoglobin.
- experience less malaise, lethargy, and tiredness episodes per 24 h.
- regain more activity tolerance after treatments.
- regain normal pulse and respiratory rates on exertion.
- regain stronger muscle/joint strength after exercise regimen.

Nursing Interventions	Rationales
Assess complaints of tiredness, fatigue, and muscle/joint weakness during activities of daily living (ADL) and usual activities; monitor vital signs.	Tiredness in RA increases over 4–5 h daily with usual activities. Increases in pulse and respirations occur due to anemia with less oxygen and red blood cells available.

Nursing Interventions	Rationales
Assist with ADL as needed.	Assistance helps conserve available energy.
Provide trapeze, assistive devices, and side rails for use.	Use of assistive devices also helps conserve energy and muscle/joint functions.
Provide uninterrupted periods of time for rest.	Persons with active RA should have a.m. and p.m. rest periods and 8–10 h sleep at night.
Collaborate with patient to schedule daily exercise and realistic activity programs.	Helps patient maintain some control and schedule helps minimize energy expenditure.
Encourage participation in active exercises and ADL as able.	Active participation helps maintain muscle/joint strength and a positive outlook.
Provide atmosphere conducive to restful sleep including quiet, relaxing music or sounds, relaxation techniques, and restriction of caffeinated foods and beverages.	Unexpected noises or loud sounds disturb the atmosphere needed for continuous sleep and rest.
Administer analgesics as prescribed when patient verbalizes need for relief of pain.	Nonnarcotic analgesics are usually prescribed for persons with RA. Pain relief eases tiredness and muscle/joint weaknesses and soreness.
Provide a diet high in iron-containing foods.	Iron-containing foods aid in regaining of normal hemoglobin levels.
Monitor laboratory data: hemoglobin and hematocrit.	Levels of hemoglobin < 12 g and hematocrit $< 30\%$ are evidences of anemia.
Teach patient foods high in iron content; provide orange juice if on iron supplements.	Foods such as dried fruits, green, leafy vegetables, liver and red meats, dried beans, and peanuts are high in iron needed to increase oxygen-carrying capacity in red blood cells. Ascorbic acid enhances iron absorption.
Teach patient ways to conserve energy, such as doing tasks in	Doing activities in stages promotes energy retention, as does using

Nursing Interventions	Rationales
stages, delegating tasks to others, gathering needed supplies prior to starting activity, and using optimal positions for activities.	optimal positions and having needed supplies readily at hand.
Teach patient and significant others to monitor vital signs if appropriate.	Knowledge of proper methods of care increases self-confidence and control.

▶ NURSING DIAGNOSIS: *Impaired Physical Mobility*

Related To joint deformity, muscle weakness, and fatigue or pain

Defining Characteristics

- One or more joints are deformed with possible subluxations, deviations (frequently ulnar deviation), presence of subcutaneous nodules limiting extensor muscle functions, pain on use, and fatigue limiting physical movements.
- Range of motion (ROM) of joints is limited by pannus formation or deformity.

Patient Outcomes

The patient will

- maintain full ROM in unaffected joints.
- regain satisfactory physical mobility after treatments.
- regain satisfactory ROM in affected joints with treatments.

Nursing Interventions	Rationales
Assess ROM of all joints, assessing affected joints last.	Assessing unaffected joints first lessens discomfort and increases cooperation.
Assess gait patterns, posture, and balance.	Gait is usually normal in RA unless hips or knees are affected, when balance and posture may also be affected.
Assist with ADL as needed according to joints affected.	In RA joints of fingers and wrists are frequently bilaterally involved and assistance is needed and

Nursing Interventions	Rationales
	welcomed if joint movements are limited.
Assist patient to positions of comfort as needed.	Frequent position changes ease discomfort of affected muscles and joints.
Assist patient to ambulate as required.	Ambulation may be slow due to lower extremity or spinal involvement and joint deformity.
Assist patient with ROM exercises as needed.	Active ROM exercises help maintain muscle strength; passive exercises also help maintain joint functions.
Collaborate with physical or occupational therapists for individualized exercise regimen and/or assistive devices as needed.	Physical therapy treatments and occupational therapy devices and strategies can help the patient with hand and wrist involvement to maintain physical muscle/joint mobility and self-care.
Encourage patient to recognize limitations and ask for assistance as needed.	Recognizing one's limitations and seeking guidance or assistance is a positive step in RA and other conditions.
Encourage patient's participation in proposed therapies such as use of paraffin baths, ice immersions, medications, rest, and other proposed treatments.	Treatments of RA are multiple and ongoing (see Table 5.1, page 82). The regimen is designed to increase mobility and ameliorate the disease process.
Use splints, rolls, or other devices to affected joints.	Assistive devices help maintain functional alignment to improve or maintain mobility.
Place necessary items within patient's reach; encourage independence.	Independence is enhanced by having readily available articles for use.
Establish a regular schedule of repositioning.	Repositioning helps maintain joint functions and lessens deleterious effects, such as development of contractures. Patients with RA tend to keep joints in a position of comfort which can lead to flexion shortening and contractures.

Nursing Interventions	Rationales
Teach patient proper use of assistive devices, splints, paraffin, ice, or medications.	Rheumatoid arthritis is a chronic disease which requires patient's understanding and compliance over time for maximal benefits.
Teach relaxation techniques; use audio tapes to enhance instructions.	Relaxation techniques lessen muscle tension and aid ROM.
Teach purpose of proper positions of all joints.	Proper positions help maintain joint mobility and lessen development of contractures.
Encourage patient to use swimming pool to exercise joints.	Joints under water lose the effects of gravity and exercise is easier and less injurious to joints.

▶ NURSING DIAGNOSIS: *Self-Care Deficit—Bathing/Hygiene, Dressing/Grooming, Feeding, and/or Toileting*

Related To disease/inflammatory involvement of fingers, hands and wrists, or other joints

Defining Characteristics

Bathing/Hygiene; Dressing/Grooming: Limited ability to

- groom self-satisfactorily
- hold or use wash cloth, towel, soap, or tooth brush in positions or for time needed
- lift or carry filled basins or glasses
- remove, reapply, or fasten clothing
- sense safe temperatures of bath or shower water

Feeding: Limited ability to

- handle silverware to cut and bring foods to mouth

Toileting: Limited ability to

- manipulate clothing for toileting
- perform proper toileting hygiene
- sit on or rise from toilet or commode

Patient Outcomes

The patient will

- achieve self-confidence and increase self-worth and self-respect while doing and completing self-care.
- develop self-care skills necessary to function in family and society.

- do self-care activities with minimal/moderate energy expenditure and minimal risk of injury.

Nursing Interventions	Rationales
Assess patient's ability to do own self-care, grooming, or toileting.	Learning exact patient abilities and/or limitations helps nurse plan or provide individualized care.
Monitor patient's current state of disease activity before encouraging more independence.	Increasing joint stress or activities during acute flares of RA may be detrimental to joints and other tissues. Use chart data, physician's comments, and patient statements to monitor current disease activity.
Assist patient with self-care grooming or toileting as needed; keep needed objects in easy reach; avoid awkward postures or stretching.	Assistance conserves energy for additional activities. Having items close prevents unsafe joint or muscle use.
Identify sources of excessive energy expenditure such as effort or length of time needed to complete activity, muscle/joint groups involved, environmental conditions.	Some self-care activities may unnecessarily tire patient or use diseased muscles/joints unnecessarily or unsafely.
Provide clothing with modified fasteners, self-adhering closures, zippers, elastic waist, or oversized neck.	Clothing modifiers ease removal or application of clothing.
Allow sufficient time for patient to perform as many bathing, dressing, and grooming activities as possible; avoid rushing patient; lay out clothing as needed.	Being as independent as possible increases patient's self-confidence and self-worth.
Provide foods best handled by patient such as finger foods, soft foods, foods in small pieces, and liquids.	Being able to feed self most foods independently maintains skills and confidence.
Assist with meal set-up as needed, such as opening containers, cutting foods into smaller pieces, putting spreads on bread, pouring liquids, and opening condiment packages.	Patients with inflamed joints and muscles have difficulty performing skills requiring dexterity and strength.
Place person in optimal position for eating such as up in a chair or high Fowler's in bed, if condition permits.	Upright positions aid chewing, deglutition, and passage of foods into stomach.

Nursing Interventions	Rationales
If needed, provide adaptive utensils, such as larger handles, splints, or longer straws or tubing.	Use of adaptive utensils conserves joint/muscle use and energy.
Provide bedside commode, urinal, or bed pan.	Use of these utensils helps conserve energy and lessens stress on inflamed joints.
Provide safety assistive devices such as raised toilet seat, grab bars, or tub seat if needed.	Safety equipment increases patient's ability to move and perform toileting activities safely.
Assist patient to open, raise, or lower clothing if needed.	Persons with acutely inflamed joints may need some assistance for toileting.
Maintain clear pathway to bathroom; keep bathroom lighted at night.	All safety measures are vital for patient care.
Praise and encourage patient's efforts to do more self-care and toileting.	Praise and encouragement recognize patient's efforts to become or maintain independence and to maintain or regain self-confidence.

▶ NURSING DIAGNOSIS: *Acute Pain*

Related To inflammatory condition of joints

Defining Characteristics

- Altered functions in one or more joints
- Deformity of one or more joints
- Edema and stiffness in one or more joints
- Increased temperature in one or more joints
- Weakened muscles or tendons in one or more joints

Patient Outcomes

The patient will

- obtain relief of pain through medications and physical therapies.
- use strategies such as audio tapes, relaxation exercises, imagery, or other diversionary activities to enhance pain relief.

Nursing Interventions	**Rationales**
Assess sites of pain, its severity, duration, and type, and other characteristics; have patient state amount of pain on a scale of 1–10 or another appropriate scale.	Having specific information related to the patient's pain helps the nurse provide the most appropriate relief measures.
Administer narcotic or nonnarcotic analgesics as prescribed.	Acute pain is usually relieved (to tolerable levels) through q4h or around the clock administration of analgesics.
Monitor patient's statements of pain relief; use flow sheet to plot progress or continued presence of pain.	Monitoring helps determine adequacy of pain relief and/or need for adjustments.
Encourage use of physical therapies such as active and passive exercises, paraffin wraps, hot or cold compresses, massage, and/or orthotic devices as needed.	These therapies help relieve inflammation and pain by increasing circulation, relieving muscle tension, and "flushing away" waste products from the site. Massage decreases muscle tension.
Encourage use of diversionary activities, music, audio tapes, imagery, or other strategies to ease pain episodes.	Such activities augment other pain relief activities for most persons.
Teach patient to record pain and activities to determine what precipitates or relieves pain.	Individual patient's reactions vary according to the specific relief activity utilized and the release of the patient's endorphins.
Teach patient/significant others side effects of narcotics and nonnarcotic analgesics.	Patients may be reluctant to take pain medications due to side effects. Side effects can usually be managed so pain relief can be maintained over time.

▶ NURSING DIAGNOSIS: *Impaired Gas Exchange*

Related To anemia and lung involvement from rheumatoid arthritis

Defining Characteristics

- Altered oxygen supply to tissues
- Decreased breath sounds
- Increased respiratory rates
- Paleness and tiredness

Patient Outcomes

The patient will

- achieve satisfactory hematocrit (40–50%) and hemoglobin (greater, equal 12 g) levels.
- regain breath sounds in all lobes.
- regain normal respiratory rates.
- regain normal skin color and relief of tiredness.

Nursing Interventions	Rationales
Assess laboratory data, chest sounds, vital signs, and other signs of respiratory functions.	These data help determine appropriate strategies to treat anemia and lung conditions.
Encourage deep breathing q4h; note color and amount of sputum expectorated.	Deep breathing is vital for total alveolar perfusion; sputum color, presence, and amount are indicative of lung inflammation or infection.
Monitor breath sounds in all lobes q4h.	Breath sounds should be heard clearly in all lobes; if not heard, blockage of ventilation must be considered.
Position patient in Fowler's or high Fowler's position for 30 min or longer, if tolerated, several times daily.	Raising the head of the bed lowers the diaphragm to aid respiratory efforts and lessen edema.
Have patient use respiratory aid (incentive spirometer) q2–4h.	Use of incentive spirometry helps increase respiratory reserve.
Observe or monitor color of conjunctiva, finger nails, and lips daily.	Paleness of named tissues is indicative of anemia, which also affects respiratory functions.
Monitor hematocrit and hemoglobin laboratory data.	These data give evidence of effects of medications to lessen anemia.
If patient has pulmonary congestion, encourage coughing; monitor amount and color of sputum produced.	Coughing aids clearing of secretions from airways; yellow or green colors of sputum are indicative of pulmonary infection.
Note signs of forgetfulness, if present.	Forgetfulness is a sign of decreased cerebral oxygenation and perfusion, secondary to anemia and impaired gas exchange.

Nursing Interventions	Rationales
Teach patient foods high in iron content.	Iron intake aids in the formation of hemoglobin and utilization of oxygen by red blood cells.

▶ NURSING DIAGNOSIS: *Sleep Pattern Disturbance*

Related To pain, muscle or joint soreness or stiffness

Defining Characteristics

- Feelings of not having restful or sufficient sleep on rising
- Frequent wakenings from sleep
- Inability to fall asleep easily or quickly at bedtime or after wakening during night

Patient Outcomes

The patient will have

- lessened muscle/joint soreness or stiffness or pain to interfere with sleep.
- long periods (6–7 h) of uninterrupted sleep.
- restful sleep after wakeful periods.

Nursing Interventions	Rationales
Assess sleep patterns during day naps and nighttime sleep.	Determining when, how often, and why wakings occur provides data to clarify extent of the problem and some possible solutions.
Monitor effects of medications that may interfere with sleep; avoid caffeine-containing liquids.	Side effects of steroid medications, commonly used in RA, include insomnia and mood swings; diuretic medications may wake patient to use bathroom; some anti-inflammatory medications cause gastric irritation which may cause pain and waken patient. Caffeine-containing liquids are stimulatory and do not promote rest.
Assist patient, if needed, to take warm bath or shower, to use heat to joints, or with sedative medications.	Warmth or heat lessens muscle/joint soreness and aids muscle relaxation to aid sleep; sedative

Nursing Interventions	Rationales
	medications lower responses to environmental stimuli to help with sleep.
Position patient flat in bed with pillows to back and between legs when on side.	A flat bed position decreases possibility of development of contractures in inflamed joints.
Offer warm milk and a snack if desired at bedtime.	Milk contains l-tryptophan, which induces sleep.
Reduce environmental noises and sounds; close curtains to darken room.	A quiet, darkened environment promotes sleep.
Administer prescribed pain or sedative medications at bedtime.	Analgesics lower pain thresholds to aid pain relief and sedatives help induce sleep.
Tighten bed linens and replace damp linens as needed.	Smooth, wrinkle-free, and dry linens lessen pressure on sore or tender tissues.
Provide time for patient to express any concerns related to RA, pain, personal or family worries, or other factors that might lead to sleep disruption.	Nighttime sometimes accentuates concerns or worries.
Assist patient to bathroom, if needed, prior to bedtime.	Rest and sleep are facilitated by having an empty bladder and preparing self for sleep.
Teach relaxation techniques that patient can use for rest at bedtime.	Achieving muscle relaxation aids patients to fall asleep more easily and promotes longer sleep periods.

▶ NURSING DIAGNOSIS: *Altered Role Performance*

Related To joint deformities, soreness, and fatigue

Defining Characteristics

- Edema, stiffness, and pain in fingers and wrists of both hands
- Unable to complete usual tasks because of weakened and deformed hands and wrists

- Subluxations, slipped tendons, and presence of Bouchard's and Heberden's nodes
- Tires quickly while attempting to complete usual tasks and role responsibilities

Patient Outcomes

The patient will
- return to usual roles and activities with treatments.
- regain functional capacities of affected muscles and joints after treatments.
- use suggested treatments, including surgery, to restore satisfactory muscle and joint functions.

Nursing Interventions	Rationales
Assess condition of fingers and wrists: bilateral presence of deformities, types of deformities, ROM of joints, and complaints of soreness, stiffness, and edema. Assess usual roles and responsibilities.	Specific data are vital for development of an individualized care plan and treatment regimen.
Assist patient to define or determine what roles are unable to be continued because of current condition.	Data help clarify limitations and possible role changes needed, either temporarily or permanently.
Assist patient to define roles in family and social network in relationship to current condition.	Data help patient and significant others determine optimal understandings and expectations.
Discuss (or clarify) proposed and on-going therapies.	Discussions clarify plans of care.
Clarify patient's understandings regarding functional changes with treatments.	Clarifications help reinforce realistic expectations.
Encourage patient to verbalize feelings related to deformities, fatigue, and chronicity of condition.	Verbalization helps patient deal with effects of disease.
Teach patient strategies to cope with physical limitations.	Learning enhances patient's strengths to cope with this chronic illness
Reiterate physician's explanations of upcoming treatments, such as synovectomies.	Synovectomy relieves inflammation for varying periods after removal and before the synovium regrows.

Nursing Interventions	Rationales
Collaborate with other health team members, such as physical and occupational therapists or social worker, for specific strategies to aid role performances.	Many strategies can be used to aid the patient's efforts to restore satisfactory muscle and joint functions.
Encourage patient's continuing prescribed medication regimen.	Rheumatoid arthritis is controlled with continued intake of many medications, as listed in Table 3.2, page 47.

► NURSING DIAGNOSIS: *Impaired Home Maintenance Management*

Related To chronicity of RA, joint deformities, fatigue and anemia, and impaired physical mobilities

Defining Characteristics

- Inability to lift, move, or carry dishes or cooking pans and other utensils
- Inability to do usual cleaning, washing, or vacuuming
- Presence of multiple healing incisional areas after synovectomies

Patient Outcomes

The patient will

- learn energy conservation techniques.
- regain many home management skills after treatments.
- regain sufficient strength and energy to manage home safely.

Nursing Interventions	Rationales
Assess effects of medical or surgical treatments on patient's usual activities in home management.	Rheumatoid arthritis affects women 3 : 1 over men. Women tend to have more home management responsibilities and activities.
Monitor effects of medications as causes of fatigue and anemia.	Steroids cause decreased collagen synthesis, causing muscle weakness and tiredness. Anemia is also a side effect of steroid medications. Anti-inflammatory medications, antibiotics, and antineoplastic

Nursing Interventions	Rationales
	medications also may lead to anemia, WBC decreases, and fatigue.
Observe patient's ability to do home management tasks with dressings or orthotic devices.	Dressings and splints interfere with normal flexing of joints. Splints may aid lifting by maintaining a more "fixed" or stable joint.
Encourage gradual increase in home activities as healing and disease control progresses.	A gradual increase in activities prevents overtiring or increase in fatigue.
Use occupational therapist's suggestions to preserve joint functions and to conserve energy; suggestions may include long-handled utensils or reachers, oversized rubber handles for knives, silverware, or other utensils, and doing some tasks in stages or after rest periods.	Using muscles and joints with aids helps conserve energy and lessens muscle/joint work efforts.
Collaborate with patient/significant others to arrange for temporary home health services, such as a home health aide or housecleaning aide.	Temporary aides help patient have time to recover from surgical treatments and to regain strength before resuming home maintenance activities.
Collaborate with therapists for continuing rehabilitative therapies in the home or outpatient setting.	Continuing such services after discharge promotes return to independence.
Teach patient to pace self in resumption of activities.	Gradual resumption promotes healing and lessens fatigue.

▶ NURSING DIAGNOSIS: *Altered Nutrition—Less Than Body Requirements*

Related To anemia and decreased intake of nutrients

Defining Characteristics

- Fatigue and tiredness
- Hemoglobin < 12 g and hematocrit < 30%
- Increased respiratory rates
- Paleness of conjunctivae, nail beds, and skin

Patient Outcomes

The patient will

- attain weight stabilization without additional losses.
- gradually regain lost weight at an average of 1 lb/3 weeks.
- regain normal appetite to increase intake of nutritious foods to 2,500 calories daily.
- regain hemoglobin and hematocrit levels within normal levels.
- regain normal skin color, conjunctivae, and nail bed colors.
- verbalize less tiredness and fatigue as intake of well-balanced diet and iron-containing foods is achieved.

Nursing Interventions	Rationales
Assess skin color, laboratory data, and complaints of fatigue and tiredness.	Individualized data help when developing a specific plan of care.
Assess food likes and dislikes in relation to dietary intake.	Anemia may be related to the disease process as well as to low intake of iron-containing foods.
Discuss decreased appetite and anemia as components of RA and medications.	Side effects of steroids include anorexia, anemia, and altered metabolism of carbohydrates, proteins, and fats.
Collaborate with dietitian to provide a well-balanced diet high in iron-containing foods.	Diet should include up to 2,500 calories with complex carbohydrates, complete proteins, and low-fat foods. Iron-containing foods include dried fruits such as raisins, green leafy vegetables, and lean red meats.
Add a dietary supplement to be taken between meals.	Supplements permit smaller meals to be eaten at mealtimes. Smaller meals are less fatiguing than three large meals.
Discuss with physician schedule of medications to lessen anorexia and gastric distress.	Medications may be given immediately after meals to lessen side effects that could occur between or before meals. Antacids also help decrease gastric irritation and distress.
Encourage patient to record foods and intake in log book or diary.	Active participation increases patient's sense of well-being and control of life.

Nursing Interventions	**Rationales**
Assist family member to plan four to six high-protein, high-calorie small meals daily; some additives can increase calorie intake, such as hot cereal with raisins and butter; yogurt with berries or nuts, or apples with peanut butter.	Assistance with food and meal preparation allows patient time to rest. Some food smells may also lessen appetite during food preparation.
Encourage patient to brush teeth and use mouth rinse before meals.	Cleaning teeth and oral tissues enhances taste and appetite.
Provide quiet environment before and after meals so patient can rest approximately 1 h before and after.	Rest helps prepare body for food intake and digestion after meals.
Teach patient how to prevent respiratory infections.	Respiratory infections increase respirations even more than already increased with anemia and fatigue.
Teach patient energy-conserving techniques and pacing of ADL.	Depending on severity of anemia and fatigue, energy must be conserved as much as possible so patient can gradually increase self-care until independence is regained.
Teach patient to gradually increase length of distances walked as food intake increases and anemia is corrected.	Exercise is vital to maintain muscle strength but must be paced to prevent undue fatigue.

▶ NURSING DIAGNOSIS: *Knowledge Deficit*

Related To diagnosis of RA, its manifestations, and its treatment regimen

Defining Characteristics

- Frequent questions or lack of questions
- Newness of diagnosis
- Unfamiliarity with disease process, its manifestations, and treatment regimen

Patient Outcomes

The patient will

- ask appropriate questions related to effects of disease on self and family or significant others.

- verbalize understanding of RA, its possible course, and its multiple treatment options after explanations and learning opportunities.

Nursing Interventions	Rationales
Assess patient's/significant others' understanding of RA, its usual course, and proposed treatment plan.	Teaching efforts must be based on patient's/significant others' level of knowledge or understanding.
Provide a quiet environment for teaching sessions.	A quiet environment with visual aids is usually optimal for teaching-learning efforts.
Use teaching techniques appropriate to patient's learning style, attention span, and ability to integrate material presented.	Learning styles vary according to age, prior learning experiences, present comfort or discomfort, unfamiliar terms, disruptions, or amount of material presented in session. Usually, use of visual aids, pictures, or charts aids learning.
Reinforce physician's explanations about RA according to patient's specific stage of disease, organ involvement and proposed medical treatment plans, exercise programs, medications, and other proposed treatments.	All explanations must be specific to the individual patient according to the symptoms and treatments proposed since there is a great variety of treatments for RA (see Table 5.1, page 82).
Reiterate the need for ongoing physician care and follow-up.	Rheumatoid arthritis has flares and remissions that may require changes in the treatment regimen to prevent development of complications or increase in deformities or other symptoms.
Review the medication protocol, expected side effects, purposes of ROM exercises, use of heat and cold therapies, orthoses, and surgical or other therapies as necessary after initial teaching.	Review helps assure correctness and completeness of information.

▶ NURSING DIAGNOSIS: *Altered Nutrition—Less Than Body Requirements*

Related To anorexia, fatigue, gastric distress, or immunosuppressive therapy

Defining Characteristics

- Anorexia secondary to side effects of medications
- Fatigue secondary to inflammatory processes or steroids
- Gastric distress secondary to anti-inflammatory medications
- Immunosuppressive effects of methotrexate such as anorexia, decreased white or red blood cells, and oral ulcerations
- Nausea or vomiting
- Weight loss

Patient Outcomes

The patient will

- have intake of high-quality foods to meet daily needs.
- regain satisfactory intake of food without marked anorexia, nausea, or vomiting.
- regain weight to within normal limits.

Nursing Interventions	Rationales
Assess food preferences according to how patient feels; include alternative food choices as able.	Lack of appetite and presence of nausea or vomiting provide a challenge to secure adequate intake of high-quality foods.
Offer oral hygiene and local oral anesthetic such as xylocaine viscous to lessen discomfort of oral lesions, if present.	Having a clean-tasting and soothed oral cavity adds to food intake.
Offer foods that are soft without harsh surfaces, neither too hot or cold nor too spicy.	Oral lesions can become more irritated by foods that are harsh, coarse, or too spicy or with temperature extremes.
Offer up to six small, frequent meals per day.	Small meals are more easily tolerated because of anorexia or gastric distress.
Encourage family to bring in favorite foods.	Eating familiar foods prepared according to specific likes gives patient a sense of control and may increase intake.
Monitor laboratory data such as hematocrit, hemoglobin, white and red blood cell counts, electrolytes, and protein levels.	These data give indications of current health condition or status, as well as indications of needed changes.

Nursing Interventions	Rationales
Monitor weights daily or as prescribed.	Daily or less frequent weighings are indicators of adequacy of intake.
Offer high-calorie or high-protein supplements between meals and at bedtime.	Such supplements increase high-quality intake.

DISCHARGE PLANNING/CONTINUITY OF CARE

- Provide written information of medication regimen and review expected side effects.
- Arrange for follow-up physician's visit.
- Establish plans for refilling prescribed medications.
- Refer to local chapter of the Arthritis Foundation for additional information or services.
- Refer to occupational and physical therapists for home maintenance and exercise regimens at home.
- Provide phone numbers and contact persons for support groups, if available in community.

Table 5.1 • Various Treatments for Rheumatoid Arthritis

Education for patient and family
Therapeutic exercises
Applications of heat and cold, often alternating
Use of orthotic devices (splints)
Occupational and physical therapies
Medications:
- Divided doses of salicylates (primarily aspirin)
- Anti-inflammatory drugs other than aspirin
- Glucocorticoids, in low or high doses
- Antineoplastic drugs
- Immunosuppressive drugs
- Antirheumatic drugs, such as gold salts and penicillamine (Cuprimine, Depen)
- Analgesic drugs

Reconstructive surgery of joints

REFERENCES

Abelson, R. (1991). The autoimmune gold rush. *Forbes, 148*(12), 198–200.

Bynum, T. E. (1989). NSAID-induced gastropathy: A gastroenterologist's point of view. *Journal of Musculoskeletal Medicine, 4*(3, Suppl.), S18–20.

Condemi, J. J. (1992). The autoimmune diseases. *Journal of the American Medical Association, 268*(20), 2882–2892.

D'Cruz, D., & Hughes, G. (1993). Rheumatoid arthritis: The clinical features. *Journal of Musculoskeletal Medicine, 8*(1), 85–95.

Diab, M. (1993). The role of type IX collagen in osteoarthritis and rheumatoid arthritis. *Orthopaedic Review, 22*(2), 165–170.

Fife, R. Z. (1993). Methotrexate use in juvenile rheumatoid arthritis. *Journal of Orthopaedic Nursing, 12*(1), 32–36.

Hicks, J. E. (1989). Exercise for patients with inflammatory arthritis. *Journal of Musculoskeletal Medicine, 6*(10), 40–56.

Kim, M. J., McFarland, G. K. & McLane, A. M. (1993). *Pocket guide to nursing diagnoses* (5th ed.). St. Louis: Mosby-Yearbook.

Kirschenbaum, D., Schneider, L. K., Adams, D. C., & Cody, R. P. (1993). Arthroplasty of the metacarpophalangeal joints with use of silicone-rubber implants in patients who have rheumatoid arthritis. Long-term results. *Journal of Bone and Joint Surgery, 75-A*(1), 3–12.

Melvin, J. L. (1989). *Rheumatic disease in the adult and child: Occupational therapy and rehabilitation* (3rd ed.). Philadelphia: Davis.

Ries, M. D., Dennis, D. A., & Clayton, M. L. (1992). Surgery in rheumatoid arthritis—the lower extremity. *Journal of Musculoskeletal Medicine, 9*(10), 29–46.

Salmond, S. W., Mooney, N. E., & Verdisco, L. A. (1991). *Core curriculum for orthopaedic nursing* (2nd ed.). Pitman, N J: Janetti

Waxman, J. (1993). Clues to differentiating between osteoarthritis and rheumatoid arthritis. *Journal of Musculoskeletal Medicine, 10*(3, Suppl.), S7–S13.

ANKYLOSING SPONDYLITIS

Ankylosing spondylitis (AS) is an inflammatory condition of the vertebral column and the sacroiliac joints. Additionally, the joints of the shoulders, hips, and knees may also be involved in later stages of the disease. The affected joints become stiff, deformed, and immovable (ankylosed).

ETIOLOGIES

- Probable genetic basis with presence of human leukocyte antigen (HLA) B27 antigen in 90% of patients
- Possible autoimmune correlation

CLINICAL MANIFESTATIONS

- Ankylosis of vertebral and sacroiliac joints with "bamboo spine" appearance
- Anterior uveitis
- Excessive thoracic kyphosis
- Forward flexion of head and neck
- Low back pain, most often beginning in sacral area with eventual obliteration of lordotic sacral curvature
- Male ratio 8 : 1 over female, with peak incidence ages 20–40
- Muscle spasms, severe at times
- Peripheral arteritis
- Urethritis

CLINICAL/DIAGNOSTIC FINDINGS

- Elevated erythrocyte sedimentation rate
- Excessive thoracic kyphosis, along with forward flexion of head and neck
- History of low back pain, especially in lumbosacral area for 3 or more months
- Physical examination of muscle tightening/spasms and pain in lumbosacral area
- Roentgenographic findings of "bamboo spine," ankylosis of vertebrae along vertebral column

▶ NURSING DIAGNOSIS: *Impaired Physical Mobility*

Related To vertebral ankyloses, kyphosis, and forward flexion of head and neck

Defining Characteristics

- Downward gaze due to forward flexion of head and neck
- Excessive thoracic kyphosis
- Fusion (ankylosis) of vertebral segments along spinal column

Patient Outcomes

The patient will

- maintain satisfactory physical mobility for many years.
- retain and regain some range of motion (ROM) of affected joints for many years.

Nursing Interventions	Rationales
Observe patient's posture and gait; note positions when standing, walking, sitting, or lying down.	Ankylosing spondylitis causes inflammation of all vertebral segments, thereby affecting both posture and gait when the hips and knees are also affected.
Encourage ROM exercises as able and to maintain exercise regimen.	Rest is contraindicated in ankylosing spondylitis as it leads to earlier ankylosis. Exercise is stressed to keep joints mobile.
Assist patient to positions of comfort; if in bed, keep bed flat to maintain extension of the vertebral column.	Pillows help the patient to maintain side-lying positions. Loss of normal lordotic curve and presence of excessive kyphosis make positioning for comfort a nursing challenge.
Offer back massage several times daily.	Massage lessens muscle tiredness and eases muscle spasms.
Encourage patient to maintain proper bed positions and to avoid lying prone.	Side lying and back lying are proper positions. The prone position lessens respiratory excursions and puts joints in more forward position (shoulders) leading to more kyphosis.
Encourage patient to do deep-breathing exercises q4h.	Deep-breathing exercises help maintain respiratory reserves which are restricted by the excessive kyphosis and joint ankylosis.

▶ NURSING DIAGNOSIS: *Body Image Disturbance and Altered Role Performance*

Related To severe kyphosis and rigidity of spine

Defining Characteristics

- Ankylosis of all spinal segments and possibly of shoulder, hip, and knee joints
- Marked fixed forward flexion of head and neck
- Persistent lumbosacral pain and muscle spasms
- Severe or excessive kyphosis

Patient Outcomes

The patient will

- experience less muscle/joint stiffness after treatments.
- retain satisfactory social interactions.
- regain a positive body image and social roles after treatments.

Nursing Interventions	Rationales
Clarify implicit or expressed concerns.	Concerns may be related to spinal rigidity, inability to look another person in the eye, or chronicity of disease, which affects patient's ability to do usual roles and activities.
Encourage compliance with treatment regimen over time (may include cervical spinal fusion and total joint replacement).	Treatments help lessen inflammatory effects of disease; surgical treatments may increase joint movements (total joint replacements) and a cervical spinal fusion allows a person to look straight ahead and overcomes forward flexion of head and neck. Continuing treatments aid in maintaining a healthier state over time.
Encourage the patient's active participation in usual roles when condition permits.	Active participation helps patient maintain socialization with family and work place personnel.
Encourage patient to participate in team recreational activities such as team or group swimming and walking.	Such participation helps maintain socialization and inclusion in activities.

▶ NURSING DIAGNOSIS: *Acute Pain*

Related To muscle spasms and joint limitations of movements

Defining Characteristics

- Acute pain in entire spinal column and other major joints
- Muscle spasms along spinal column
- Spondylitis leading to marked limitation of movements in spinal movements and other major joints

Patient Outcomes

The patient will

- experience relief of pain and muscle spasms with medications.
- have increased joint use after treatments.

Nursing Interventions	Rationales
Assess patient for the presence, amount, severity, sites, duration, and type of pain.	These data are vital for individualized plan of care.
Administer analgesic and anti-inflammatory medications as prescribed; monitor effects of medications to relieve pain.	Relief of painful muscle spasms is a major goal.
Monitor effects of warm, moist compresses to painful joints.	Warm, moist compresses increase circulation and aid removal of wastes to lessen pain and muscle spasms.
Massage back several times daily.	Massage relaxes painful muscles to lessen spasms.
Observe patient's movements when changing positions.	Observations may provide evidence of easier movements, continued pain and stiffness, or only moderate relief. Changes in medications may be required.
Encourage back-lying or side-lying positions with use of pillows for support.	Proper positions and use of pillows helps prevent additional trauma.
Listen for complaints of side effects of medications, such as gastric irritation or distress, gastrointestinal bleeding, mood swings, anemia, diarrhea, or constipation.	Steroid medications have multiple side effects which can lead to need to change medications.

▶ NURSING DIAGNOSIS: *Knowledge deficit*

Related To newness or suddenness of diagnosis of AS

NOTE: For defining characteristics, patient outcomes, and nursing interventions, refer to Rheumatoid Arthritis on page 63–83.

DISCHARGE PLANNING/CONTINUITY OF CARE

- Refer to physical therapists for home exercise regimen.
- Refer to home care nurses for follow-up wound care, nutritional assistance, or assistance with activities of daily living.
- Arrange for follow-up physician's visit.
- Review medication regimen and expected side effects; provide written guidelines.

REFERENCES

Burke, M. M., & Walsh, M. B. (1992). *Gerontologic nursing.* St. Louis: Mosby-Yearbook.

Hogstel, M. O. (1992). *Clinical manual of gerontological nursing.* St. Louis: Mosby-Yearbook.

Kaplan, P. E., & Tanner, E. D. (1989). *Musculoskeletal pain and disability* Norwalk, CT: Appleton & Lange.

Khan, M. A., Lai, J. H., Chou, C. T., Chang, D. M., & Liu, H. C. (1993). Recognizing and managing fractures in ankylosing spondylitis. *Journal of Musculoskeletal Medicine, 8*(1), 45–57.

Kim, M. J., McFarland, G. K., & McLane, A. M. (1993). *Pocket guide to nursing diagnoses* (5th ed.). St. Louis: Mosby-Yearbook.

Lewis, S. M., & Collier, I. C. (1992). *Medical-surgical nursing assessment and management of clinical problems* (3rd ed.). St. Louis: Mosby-Yearbook.

SYSTEMIC LUPUS ERYTHEMATOSUS

Systemic lupus erythematosus (SLE) is an autoimmune disease that affects all collagen-containing connective tissues in the body including the tissues around joints, the heart, lungs, kidneys, and skin. A milder form called discoid lupus erythematosus affects primarily the skin, producing a patchy red rash over parts of the skin surfaces. However, SLE is a chronic, life-shortening disease that can be treated but not cured.

ETIOLOGIES

- Autoimmune condition of collagen-containing tissues
- Environmental influences including ultraviolet light, stress, and viral infection; drug-induced SLE also occurs
- Genetic predisposition with familial clusters
- Human leukocyte antigen (HLA) DR2 and DR3 histocompatibility complexes present

CLINICAL MANIFESTATIONS

- Activation of complement leading to inflammation and destruction of cells or basement membranes
- Alternating periods of remission and exacerbation
- Decreased T-suppressor cells
- Diminished interleukin-2 production
- Fever, weight loss, extreme fatigue
- Production of autoantibodies against cellular antigens (cell nuclear antigens, cytoplasmic antigens, blood cell surface antigens)
- Variable severity from mild to rapidly progressive disease
- Malar or butterfly rash

CLINICAL/DIAGNOSTIC FINDINGS

Person is considered to have SLE if four or more of the following are present (Lewis & Collier, 1992):

- Antinuclear antigen
- Arthritis: nonerosive, involvement of two or more joints
- Discoid rash
- Hematologic disorder: hemolytic anemia, leukopenia, lymphopenia, or thrombocytopenia
- Immunologic disorder: positive lupus cell preparation; antibodies to native DNA or antibody to Sm nuclear antigen*; false-positive serologic test for syphilis
- Malar rash (over nose and cheeks)
- Neurologic disorder: seizures or psychosis
- Oral ulcers
- Photosensivitity
- Renal disorders: proteinuria or cellular casts
- Serositis: pleuritis or pericarditis

Additionally, clinical findings may include

- abnormal pulmonary function studies.
- alopecia with diffuse or patchy hair loss.
- increased susceptibility to infection.
- Raynaud phenomenon of digits or toes: pattern of whitening, cyanosis, and redness.

▶ NURSING DIAGNOSIS: *Impaired Skin Integrity*

Related To skin rash, photosensitivity, or alopecia

Defining Characteristics

- Alopecia: may be diffuse or patchy
- Photosensitivity
- Rash: may be discoid over body or mainly over nose and cheeks (butterfly rash)

Patient Outcomes

The patient will

- have no (or very few) episodes of photosensitivity reactions.
- have regression of rash over time after treatments.
- regrow lost hair.

**Anti-Sm antibody, an antibody to the Smith nuclear antigen, is a definitive serologic marker for SLE which is not demonstrated in other rheumatic diseases (Lewis & Collier, 1992).*

Nursing Interventions	Rationales
Monitor sites, color, and progression or regression of rash.	Remission and/or exacerbation of rash is one evidence of disease activity.
Administer prescribed medications: may include nonsteroidal anti-inflammatory, antimalarial, corticosteroid, or immunosuppressive medications.	Systemic lupus erythematosus can only be controlled not cured at the present time. Multiple drug therapies are used.
Apply or teach patient to apply topical ointments or sun screens as prescribed.	Ointments prevent skin ulcerations and sun screens lessen photosensitive reactions.
Discuss wearing of sun hats, long-sleeved shirts, blouses, or jackets, and long pants along with sun screens when unable to avoid being in sunlight.	Clothing prevents exposure to ultraviolet rays, as do sun screens of high protective factor (above 15 SPF).
Teach patient to keep skin clear and dry.	Patient is already susceptible to infection. Keeping the skin clean and dry helps prevent infections.
Discuss wearing of turbans, scarves, or wigs during periods of greater hair loss.	Covering hair loss helps patient's self-esteem and body image.

▶ NURSING DIAGNOSIS: *Activity Intolerance*

Related To arthralgia, muscle weakness, and fatigue

Defining Characteristics

- Acutely painful joints
- Dyspnea on exertion
- Increased pulse rates and respiratory rates on exertion
- Marked tiredness, muscle weakness and fatigue
- Unwillingness to participate in ambulation and other physical activities

Patient Outcomes

The patient will

- experience less muscle/joint soreness after range of motion (ROM) exercises.
- learn to pace self-activities to avoid dyspnea and increased pulse or respiratory rates (return to usual rates after brief rest).
- participate satisfactorily in activities to prevent problems in immobility.

Nursing Interventions	Rationales
Monitor and listen to patient's expressions of tiredness, fatigue, joint soreness, or pain before, during, and after physical activities.	Observing patient's responses and reactions is vital for changes to be implemented in the care plans.
Allow rest period before and after physical activities.	Rest periods help restore energy levels for physical activities to levels of tolerance.
Collaborate with patient to pace and set activity schedules.	Input gives the patient a sense of control within environment.
Monitor vital signs before, during, and after physical activities.	Data are indications of patient's abilities to do activities or need for more rest or less activity if vital signs show marked upward changes.
Encourage patient to lessen activities during exacerbation of disease; then gradually increase activities as acute symptoms abate.	Energy is needed during exacerbation to overcome the new symptoms; thus limited energy remains for other physical activities.
Collaborate with physical therapist to provide ROM exercises to unaffected joints; encourage use of assistive devices as needed.	Range-of-motion exercises help maintain strength of muscles; assistive devices lessen energy expenditure and prevent overuse of weakened muscles or joints.
Provide bedrest during exacerbation of SLE.	Bedrest decreases metabolism and conserves energy for vital activities.

▶ NURSING DIAGNOSIS: *Body Image Disturbance*

Related To changes in physical appearance

Defining Characteristics

- Alopecia
- Development of moon facies
- Edema
- Erythematous rash
- Purpura or petechiae
- Seizures or disorientation
- Urticaria

Patient Outcomes

The patient will

- participate actively in self-care, hygiene, and grooming.
- express positive feelings and comments about self.

Nursing Interventions	Rationales
Listen to patient's expressions of physical appearance related to manifestations of SLE and/or side effects of steroids (moon facies, purpura, petechiae, and others).	Clarifying patient's understandings helps the nurse provide individualized care.
Discuss realistic expectations related to physical appearance and changes with remission and medications.	Having realistic, factual information helps the patient gradually accept self.
Encourage self-participation in bathing, hygiene, and grooming; encourage use of cosmetics, scarves, turbans, wigs, hosiery, and clothing to cover dry lesions.	Self-participation and utilization of cosmetic aids increase the patient's positive perceptions of self.
Discuss seizure activity and control measures (medications) if prescribed or needed; discuss safety measures.	Seizures can usually be controlled with medications. Safety measures prevent injury during seizure activity.

▶ NURSING DIAGNOSIS: *Acute Pain*

Related To arthralgia and disease process (Raynaud phenomenon)

Defining Characteristics

- Arthralgia in one or more joints
- Raynaud phenomenon: whitening, bluing (cyanosis), and reddening of digits or toes

Patient Outcomes

The patient will

- experience satisfactory pain relief with analgesics.
- have decreasing episodes of Raynaud phenomenon.

Nursing Interventions	Rationales
Monitor patient's complaints of sites, extent, type, amount, and duration of joint pain.	Pain may be dull, aching, or sharp and acute, affecting one or more joints, with short periods or over long periods of day and night.

Nursing Interventions	Rationales
Administer prescribed analgesics "around the clock"; monitor effects of analgesics.	Around-the-clock administration helps maintain therapeutic blood levels for optimal analgesia and pain control.
Apply hot or cold compresses to affected joints.	Hot or cold compresses ease inflammation, lessen pain, and decrease edema (see Table 3.1, page 45, for effects of heat and cold).
Provide rest periods after pain medications are administered.	Rest permits the patient to experience optimal benefits from the analgesic medications.
Administer medications (steroids or vasodilating drugs) as prescribed to control episodes of Raynaud phenomenon.	Inflammation of small peripheral arteries is one cause of Raynaud phenomenon. Stress response may be another cause. Steroids lessen episodes as inflammation lessens. Vasodilator drugs increase steady arterial inflow.

▶ NURSING DIAGNOSIS: *Fatigue*

Related To inflammatory process of SLE

Defining Characteristics

- Extreme tiredness and fatigue
- Inability to carry out usual routines and responsibilities
- Lack of energy

Patient Outcomes

The patient will

- express being less tired or fatigued.
- express having more energy.
- have enough energy to complete priority activities.

Nursing Interventions	Rationales
Discuss patient's usual routines and responsibilities; help patient develop priorities for doing activities.	The patient's energy level will help determine which activities will have priority if all cannot be done.

Nursing Interventions	Rationales
Discuss energy conservation methods, such as sitting rather than standing, lowering work levels to avoid holding arms and hands above trunk level, when possible.	Sitting uses less muscle actions, thus less energy. Holding arms and hands above chest level takes more energy than keeping arms and hands lower, as when shelling peas or cutting beans.
Discuss resting between activities and spacing groups of activities.	Rest periods help restore energy. Spacing between activities allows time for muscle energy restoration.
Teach relaxation and stress reduction techniques.	Such exercises help muscles relax to reduce tension and help restore energy. Visualization, imagery, yoga, and medication are valuable for relaxation and stress reduction.
Teach patient symptoms of SLE exacerbation and what to report to physician; encourage on-going medical visits.	Anergy and extreme tiredness may be a sign of SLE exacerbation that should be reported to the physician. Some tiredness, however, is expected because of the inflammatory nature of SLE.

▶ NURSING DIAGNOSIS: *Knowledge Deficit*

Related To diagnosis of SLE

Defining Characteristics

- Asks frequent questions or lacks questions
- Concerned about need for multiple tests for diagnosis
- Unfamiliar with term "systemic lupus erythematosus"

Patient Outcomes

The patient will

- ask appropriate questions about effects of disease on self and family.
- verbalize understanding of need for multiple tests and meaning of terms after explanation.

Nursing Interventions	Rationales
Assess patient's level of understanding or knowledge of SLE, its course, and its treatments.	Clarifying patient's knowledge level provides the basis for teaching efforts.

Nursing Interventions	Rationales
Provide an environment conducive to learning.	A quiet area with visual aids such as pictures or charts is usually optimal for education.
Keep teaching sessions appropriate to patient's learning style, attention span, and ability to integrate material presented.	Learning styles may be verbal, visual, or written; attention may drift due to discomfort, unfamiliar terms, disruptions from family members or others, or if too much information is presented.
Reiterate physician's explanations related to SLE according to patient's specific organ involvement and proposed medical plan of treatment, exercise programs, and medications.	Because of diversity of SLE symptoms and organ involvement, explanations must be specific to the individual patient.

DISCHARGE PLANNING/CONTINUITY OF CARE

- Arrange for follow-up physician's visit.
- Provide written list of medications, their purposes, and expected side effects; review as needed for patient's understanding.
- Provide information regarding support groups of SLE in community.
- Refer to local lupus chapter for additional information or services.
- Refer to home care agency for ongoing follow-up as needed.

REFERENCES

Gulanick, M., Klopp, A., & Galanes, S. (Eds.). (1991). *Nursing care plans, nursing diagnosis, and interventions.* St. Louis: Mosby-Yearbook

Halverson, P. B., & Holmes, S. B. (1993). Systemic lupus erythematosus: Medical and nursing treatments. *Journal of Orthopaedic Nursing, 12*(1), 17–24.

Kaine, J. L., & Kahl, L. E. (1992). Which laboratory tests are useful in diagnosing SLE? *Journal of Musculoskeletal Medicine, 7*(11), 15–27.

Lewis, S. M., & Collier, L. C. (1992). *Medical-surgical nursing assessment and management of clinical problems* (3rd ed.). St. Louis: Mosby-Yearbook.

Mourad, L. A., & Droste, M. M. (1993). *The nursing process in the care of adults with orthopaedic conditions* (3rd ed.). Albany: Delmar.

Salmond, S. W., Mooney, N. E., & Verdisco, L. A. (1991). *Core curriculum for orthopaedic nursing* (2nd ed.). Pitman, NJ: Janetti.

SYSTEMIC SCLEROSIS

Systemic sclerosis (SS) (formerly called scleroderma) is a connective tissue disorder that is characterized by degenerative, fibrotic, and inflammatory changes in the skin, skeletal muscles, internal organs, blood vessels, and synovium. Its cardinal signs are skin thickening and tightening. A variant of systemic sclerosis is called CREST syndrome, noted by *C*alcinosis, *R*aynaud phenomenon, *E*sophageal hypomotility, *S*clerodactyly (harding of skin of fingers), and *T*elangiectasis (angiomas on skin). Systemic sclerosis affects women 15 : 1 over men during childbearing years.

ETIOLOGIES

- Exact etiology unclear
- May have an immunologic basis as noted below

CLINICAL MANIFESTATIONS

- Decreased skin elasticity
- Dysphagia due to esophageal hypomotility
- Malignant hypertension
- Myocardial fibrosis leading to congestive heart failure
- Painless, symmetrical swelling and thickening of skin of hands and fingers
- Platelet aggregation; can lead to ulcerations or gangrene
- Polyarthralgia
- Raynaud phenomenon plus numbness and tingling of fingers
- Renal disease
- Skin thickening and tightening; skin becomes taut and shiny

CLINICAL/DIAGNOSTIC FINDINGS

- Anticentromere antibody, marked specificity for CREST syndrome
- CREST syndrome includes elevated serum calcium levels, arterial vasospasms, hardened skin tissues, and skin angiomas
- Elevated erythrocyte sedimentation rate
- Expressionless facies with tightly pursed lips
- Presence of antinuclear antibodies (ANA) in majority of patients

- Pulmonary fibrosis
- Skin changes as given above

▶ NURSING DIAGNOSIS: *Impaired Physical Mobility*

Related To sclerotic changes in skin, arthralgia, and joint stiffness

Defining Characteristics

- Difficulty moving from place to place
- Limited range of motion (ROM) of affected joints
- Skin sclerosis, shiny and taut skin

Patient Outcomes

The patient will

- experience CREST syndrome leading to milder disease.
- live long periods without pulmonary, cardiac, or renal complications.

Nursing Interventions	Rationales
Assess specific signs of SS in patient.	Because of variable disease process, patient may have CREST or more severe manifestations of SS.
Observe patient's posture and gait.	Joints and skin are often very tight, with joint swelling, stiffness, and polyarthralgias noted. Flexion contractures and atrophy of soft tissue may be present.
Encourage ROM exercises as able; collaborate with physical therapists for exercise programs and regimen.	Exercises help muscles retain strength and functions.
Consult with occupational therapists for assistance in managing functional abilities at home or employment setting.	Guidance fosters the patient's maintaining independence.
Administer medications as prescribed; observe for side effects.	Medications may include anti-inflammatory, vasodilator, antihypertensive, or antigout medications; side effects for many drugs are given in Table 3.2, page 47.
Assist patient to ambulate, if needed.	Patient may be stiff and unsteady when rising or walking.
Observe patient for progressive symptoms of SS.	Systemic sclerosis has a variable course (see next nursing diagnosis).

▶ NURSING DIAGNOSIS: *High Risk for Additional Injury*

Risk Factors

- Abdominal distension leading to bowel obstruction
- Dysphagia
- Gastric reflux and heartburn
- Raynaud phenomenon: periods of blanching, blueness, and redness of digits, in that order
- Weight loss

Patient Outcomes

The patient will

- be relieved of Raynaud occurrences with medications.
- experience only mild esophageal problems amenable to use of antacids and soft foods.
- maintain low normal body weight.
- retain satisfactory bowel function.

Nursing Interventions	Rationales
Observe patient for presence of any of above patterns.	Patient may have one or more depending on variability of SS.
Ask patient about bowel movements; check abdominal girths daily and listen for bowel sounds every shift.	The patient should have a bowel movement at least q1–2 days, with soft, formed stool. An increasing abdominal girth may signify the beginning of a bowel obstruction. Bowel sounds or peristaltic rushes should be heard clearly in abdominal quadrants. Normally rushes occur approximately every 30 s to 1 min to propel contents to rectum.
Discuss food likes and dislikes; provide a diet of soft foods and sufficient liquids to aid deglutition; respond to complaints of gastric distress and heartburn.	Because of esophageal hypomotility, one of the hallmarks of SS, foodstuffs may lodge in lower esophagus, leading to gastric reflux and heartburn. These symptoms are treated with antacids. Soft foods with adequate fluid intake aid passage of foods into stomach.

Nursing Interventions	Rationales
Observe patient's ability to open mouth sufficiently to move food into mouth.	Some persons with SS have marked decrease in the ability to open the mouth because of skin tightening of face and mouth.
Note occurrences of Raynaud phenomenon, extent of involvement of digits or toes, and return of circulation.	Raynaud is a condition of paroxysmal vasospasms of the fingertips or toes that occurs in about 98% of persons with SS. Severe SS with repetitive Raynaud episodes can lead to gangrene of the fingertips or toes. Ulcerations may be treated with soaks and bacterial ointments.
Administer calcium channel blocker (nifedipine, diltiazem), if prescribed, for treating Raynaud phenomenon.	Calcium channel blocking drugs lessen arterial vasospasms as well as help treat the calcinosis of SS.
Stress oral hygiene and dental visits, if needed.	If oral opening is markedly decreased, it may become very difficult for the patient to do thorough brushing and care of gingivae.
Seek consultation with mental health practitioner, if needed.	Persons with SS may need assistance in dealing with body image changes, self-concept, sexuality, limited life expectancy, or other problems.

▶ NURSING DIAGNOSIS: *Knowledge Deficit*

Related To newness of diagnosis, severity of disease, or other concerns

Defining Characteristics

- Appearance of CREST syndrome
- Changes in skin, physical appearance, and other symptoms

Patient Outcomes

The patient will

- accept diagnosis after explanation and discussion of treatment options.
- accept uncertainty of disease process.

Nursing Interventions	Rationales
Reiterate or clarify physician's explanations.	The patient may not fully hear or understand physician's initial explanations because of stress or unfamiliarity with SS. Repeated explanations may be needed for more patient understanding.
Arrange a quiet environment for teaching session.	A quiet environment is more conducive to learning because of less distraction or "noise."
Use pictures or diagrams as needed to clarify explanations.	Some patients learn better through visual rather than verbal stimuli or messages.
Include family/significant others in teaching session.	Including pertinent others in sessions provides the important persons with the same information.
Explain the need for the patient to have ongoing physician care.	Systemic sclerosis may have a variable course, and complications can possibly be prevented by ongoing care.

DISCHARGE PLANNING/CONTINUITY OF CARE

- Refer to home care agency for follow-up wound and skin care as needed.
- Review medication purposes and expected side effects; provide written guidelines.
- Refer to local systemic sclerosis or arthritis chapter, as needed for additional information.
- Refer to physical therapists for prescribed exercise regimen follow-up.

Clinical Clip

A more benign form of systemic sclerosis is identified by the acryonym CREST, with each letter representing one of five common symptoms:

C = calcinosis

R = Raynaud phenomenon

E = esophageal hypomotility

S = sclerodactyly (hardening of skin of fingers)

T = telangiectasia (skin angiomas)

REFERENCES

Gulanick, M., Klopp, A., & Galanes, S. (Eds.). (1991). *Nursing care plans, nursing diagnosis, and interventions.* St. Louis: Mosby-Yearbook.

Kim, M. J., McFarland, G. K., & McLane, A. M. (1993). *Pocket guide to nursing diagnoses* (5th ed.). St. Louis: Mosby-Yearbook.

Mourad, L. A., & Droste, M. M. (1993). *The nursing process in the care of adults with orthopaedic conditions* (3rd ed.). Albany: Delmar.

Talal, N. (1992). With Sjogren syndrome, look for scleroderma. *Journal of Musculoskeletal Medicine,* 7(12), 15–16.

BURSITIS

Bursitis is inflammation of a bursa. Bursae are small sacs located near joints in muscles, tendons, or ligaments filled with synovial fluid. They lubricate the tissues in which they are contained. They can become inflamed.

ETIOLOGIES

- Excessive trauma
- Excessive friction
- Rheumatoid arthritis

CLINICAL MANIFESTATIONS

- Area of redness and tenderness around joint
- Calcification of bursa, occasionally
- Exquisite pain or tenderness near joint
- Limitation of movement of joint/muscles
- Point tenderness

CLINICAL/DIAGNOSTIC FINDINGS

- History of repetitive trauma
- Limitation of movement of tissues in affected area
- Point tenderness
- Roentgenograms may show calcified bursa

▶ NURSING DIAGNOSIS: *Acute Pain*

Related To inflamed bursa

Defining Characteristics

- Inability to use affected part without pain
- Point tenderness in bursal area
- Swelling around bursa (not always present)

Patient Outcomes

The patient will

- have resolution of the bursal inflammation.
- not develop calcifications in the bursa.

Nursing Interventions	Rationales
Assess area of pain or tenderness for edema, redness, hot area, limitation of motion, point tenderness, or other symptoms.	Bursitis usually shows common signs of inflammation and limitation of motion.
Listen to patient's complaints of pain when moves affected part(s).	Pain is usually the first sign of bursitis, with point tenderness (patient can point to spot of most pain) a common sign. The joints involved most commonly with their bursae include the shoulder and its subdeltoid and subacromial bursae, the elbow and olecranon bursa, the knee and its anserine bursa, and the trochanter and trochanteric bursa.
Note limitations of movements of affected area.	Patient verbalizes that certain movements cause most pain.
Apply moist compresses to area.	Moist compresses increase circulation to relieve inflammation.
Position, and reposition, as comfortably as possible.	Positioning relieves strain on inflamed tissues.
Administer prescribed analgesics or anti-inflammatory medications as prescribed.	These medications relieve pain and inflammation.
Assist with injection of corticosteroid into site, if done; explain increase in pain after injection.	Corticosteroids decrease inflammation and relieve pain. There is a temporary increase in pain after injection that may last 8–12 h due to the increased pressure of fluid in an enclosed space.
Support inflamed tissues and joints; handle gently.	Gentle handling lessens stress and prevents additional trauma.
Monitor effects of analgesics and corticosteroid injection.	Learning effects of treatments may indicate need for change.

▶ NURSING DIAGNOSIS: *Impaired Physical Mobility*

Related to inflamed bursa and surrounding tissues

Defining Characteristics

- Limitation of joint/muscle movements
- Redness, heat, edema, and tenderness of inflamed area

Patient Outcomes

The patient will

- experience relief (resolution) of inflammation.
- regain full range of motion (ROM) of affected tissues.

Nursing Interventions	Rationales
Assess bursal area and surrounding tissues for ROM and limitations of movements.	Data give indications of extent of inflammation for planning care.
Assist with ROM exercises as needed.	Range-of-motion exercises help maintain, retain, or regain functions of inflamed tissues.
Apply moist compresses to inflamed area.	Compresses hasten resolution of inflammation through increasing circulation to remove wastes.
Put arm in sling if shoulder bursae are inflamed; apply elastic bandages, if appropriate.	External supports decrease strain on affected joints and give support to the joints.
Monitor effects of medications and treatments on resolution of infection.	Data may indicate need to continue treatments or to add new ones.
Caution patient to avoid activities that could prevent healing of present inflammation or cause a recurrence.	Recurrence can lead to chronic inflammatory processes that can restrict or cause permanent damage.
Suggest use of pads or step stool to lessen pressure or strain on frequently used joints.	Using a pad when kneeling lessens strain on inflamed tissues (anserine bursa); use of a step stool prevents excessive pressure on shoulder bursae when lifting or reaching high shelves.

▶ NURSING DIAGNOSIS: *Knowledge Deficit*

Related To unfamiliar terms or treatments

Defining Characteristics

- Hearing terms such as subacromial or subdeltoid or anserine bursa
- Restrictions imposed by inflammatory processes

Patient Outcome

The patient will

- develop understanding of new terms through teaching and learning.
- verbalize purposes of treatments to relieve inflammation and strain on joints.

Nursing Interventions	Rationales
Assess patient's knowledge of terms: bursitis, bursa, anserine, subacromial or subdeltoid, compresses, sling, and such.	Learning what patient knows or understands is the basis for additional teaching.
Clarify the purposes and sites of bursae by use of pictures or anatomic drawings.	Using pictures or drawings enhances patient's learning.
Explain why injection of corticosteroid increases pain temporarily.	Injecting fluid into the bursal sac increases pressure in the enclosed sac (space), thereby increasing pain temporarily, which is relieved as the steroid is absorbed and inflammation is relieved.
Teach patient to curtail activities until inflammation is resolved and to use pads or supports to affected areas.	Resolution may take 4–6 weeks. Pads, sling, elastic wraps, and stools lessen strain on tender tissues.

DISCHARGE PLANNING/CONTINUITY OF CARE

- Arrange for follow-up physician's visit.
- Refer to physical therapist for exercise regimen and heat/cold therapy as prescribed.
- Review purposes of corticosteroid medication, decreasing dosages, and expected side effects; provide written guidelines.

REFERENCES

Mourad, L. A., & Droste, M. M. (1993). *The nursing process in the care of adults with orthopaedic conditions* (3rd ed.). Albany: Delmar.

Mourad, L. A. (1991). *Orthopedic disorders.* St. Louis: Mosby-Yearbook.

Walker, L. G., & Meals, R. A. (1989). Tendinitis: A practical approach to diagnosis and management. *Journal of Musculoskeletal Medicine,* 6(5), 24–54.

EPICONDYLITIS OR TENOSYNOVITIS

Epicondylitis is inflammation of the tendons where they insert in condyles of bones. Tenosynovitis is inflammation of the tendon-covering sheath around one or more tendons. Lateral epicondylitis is commonly called "tennis elbow"; medial epicondylitis is known as "golfer's elbow."

ETIOLOGIES

- Microtraumatic changes from tearing or bleeding into site

CLINICAL MANIFESTATIONS

- Edema at site around epicondyle
- Pain along tendon sheath
- Pain at epicondylar area
- Point tenderness

CLINICAL/DIAGNOSTIC FINDINGS

- Calcification at origin of tendon
- History of repetitive motions of affected extremity
- Inflamed area around epicondyle
- Scarring
- Sensory changes
- Thickening of tendon sheath

▶ NURSING DIAGNOSIS: *Impaired Physical Mobility*

Related To microtrauma to medial or lateral epicondyles, or tendon sheaths

Defining Characteristics

- Repetitive motions of affected extremity causing bleeding, scarring, and vascularity in area
- Signs of inflammation: edema, redness, pain, change in function, point tenderness; occasionally, numbness or tingling; limited range of motion (ROM)

Patient Outcome

The patient will

- regain full functions and ROM after treatments.
- retain some functions during inflammatory period.

Nursing Interventions	Rationales
Assess site for signs of inflammation: 1. For lateral epicondylitis, assess for presence of pain, point tenderness, and changes when pronates or supinates forearm on lateral side of forearm (lateral epicondylar area). Tennis swings may cause reproduction of pain, as can scaling a fish. 2. For medial epicondylitis, assess for pain and point tenderness in medial epicondylar area of forearm; may also have edema or heat; golf swing causes reproduction of pain. 3. For tenosynovitis, assess for weakness, and at times sensory changes, in specific affected tendon, as e.g., • patellar tenosynovitis: pain around top of knee when running, jumping, or climbing steps • Achilles tendinitis: nagging pain in heel when walking or running; may have edema of foot/heel • bicipital tendinitis: increasing pain in front of shoulder when reaching overhead • flexor tendinitis: cannot straighten out finger and has pain when trying to do so • gluteus maximus tendinitis: pain in hip and outside area of thigh	Each "itis" shows signs of inflammation when used by patient.

Nursing Interventions	Rationales
Discuss rationale for rest to affected part or tissues and to avoid activities that cause symptoms to recur.	Rest allows inflamed tissues to begin healing and the inflammation to resolve.
Administer analgesic or nonsteroidal anti-inflammatory medication as prescribed.	These medications decrease perception of pain plus help resolve inflammation.
Assist with injection of corticosteroid into area; explain temporary increase in pain.	Steroids help decrease inflammation. Increased pain results from increased fluid in an enclosed space.
Arrange consultation with physical therapist for prescribed exercises.	Exercises retain and regain muscles' functions as well as strengthen weakened tissues.
Teach patient how to apply hot and cold applications, if to be used.	Heat increases circulation, whereas cold decreases blood flow, and lessens pressure on inflamed nerve endings to lessen pain. Heat and cold applications can be used alternately.
Teach patient how to apply splint, immobilizer, or other orthosis, as prescribed.	Such devices ease strain on inflamed tissues, aid healing, and relieve pain.

▶ NURSING DIAGNOSIS: *Knowledge Deficit*

Related To unfamiliar terms

Defining Characteristics

- Hearing of restrictions
- Hearing unfamiliar terms such as Achilles tendinitis, lateral epicondylitis, or de Quervain tendinitis

Patient Outcomes

The patient will

- be able to explain the specific condition after a teaching session.
- verbalize purposes of treatments and rest to affected part.

Nursing Interventions	Rationales
Assess patient's understanding of his or her conditions, their cause, and the proposed treatment.	These data show the current level of patient's knowledge.
Use anatomic drawings or pictures to clarify specific location of patient's condition.	Visual aids facilitate patient's learning.
Explain purposes and effects of corticosteroid injections, if used.	Corticosteroids may be injected for anti-inflammatory effects. They may temporarily increase pain as they reinject into a "closed" area at the epicondylar area.
Clarify the need to curtail or restrict activities that led to inflammation initially.	Inflammatory changes resolve, usually, in 4–6 weeks.

DISCHARGE PLANNING/CONTINUITY OF CARE

- Complete referral to physical therapist for home care exercise regimen.
- Provide prescriptions for medications for continuous medication administration; review side effects of medications.
- Make a return-to-physician appointment.

REFERENCES

Kim, M. J., McFarland, G. K., & McLane, A. M. (1993). *Pocket guide to nursing diagnoses* (5th ed.). St. Louis: Mosby-Yearbook.

Mourad, L. A., & Droste, M. M. (1993). *The nursing process in the care of adults with orthopaedic conditions* (3rd ed.). Albany: Delmar.

Salmond, S. W., Mooney, N. E., & Verdisco, L. A. (1991). *Core curriculum for orthopaedic nursing* (2nd ed.). Pitman, NJ: Janetti.

Walker, L. G., & Meals, R. A. (1989). Tendinitis: A practical approach to diagnosis and management. *Journal of Musculoskeletal Medicine, 6*(5), 24–54.

Metabolic Diseases of Bone

Bone formation and resorption depend on adequate intake, absorption, and utilization of proteins, vitamins, calcium, and phosphorus. Imbalances in one or more of these critical areas can result in reduction of bone mass.

OSTEOMALACIA

Osteomalacia is a condition of decalcification and softening of bones in adults caused by a vitamin D deficiency. In children, the condition is called rickets.

ETIOLOGIES

- Chronic diarrhea causing loss of calcium, leading to inadequate vitamin D absorption
- Gastrointestinal malabsorption
- Lack of exposure to sunlight, needed to convert vitamin D into its absorbable form
- Pregnancy with inadequate intake of vitamin D and calcium
- Renal disease with increased losses of calcium and/or phosphorus

CLINICAL MANIFESTATIONS

- Fractures of bones
- Persistent skeletal pain
- Progressive deformities of bones of extremities and spine
- Progressive muscle weakness

CLINICAL/DIAGNOSTIC FINDINGS

- Decreased serum levels of calcium and phosphorus
- Diagnostic of osteomalacia: Presence of Looser zones on x-ray films. These zones are areas of decalcification in bones
- Elevated serum alkaline phosphatase
- Roentgenograms show generalized bone demineralization and multiple bone deformities

▶ NURSING DIAGNOSIS: *Impaired Physical Mobility*

Related To bone decalcification and bone deformities and possible fractures

Defining Characteristics

- Deformities of limbs; abnormal spinal curvatures
- Fractures of one or more bones

Patient Outcomes

The patient will

- regain normal serum levels of calcium, phosphorus, and alkaline phosphatase.
- regain normal bone structure.
- increase intake and utilization of vitamin D and calcium.
- regain normally shaped bones and posture after treatments.

Nursing Interventions	Rationales
Assess posture and gait; note ability to walk with or without aid.	Patient may have abnormal posture and gait due to bone deformities, muscle weakness, or fracture.
Note ability to walk requested distances.	May be able to walk only short distances because of muscle weakness or skeletal pain.
Check bony prominences for signs of pressure or presence of sores or ulcerations.	May place weight on bony prominences because of deformed bones. Clothing or shoes may rub abnormally and cause soreness or ulcerations.

▶ NURSING DIAGNOSIS: *High Risk for Injury (Fracture)*

Risk Factors

- Deformed bones through body
- Weak bones due to demineralization

Patient Outcomes

The patient will

- have decreased risk of fracture after treatments.
- regain normally shaped bones and improved posture after treatments.

Nursing Interventions	Rationales
Assess shape of bones throughout body; assess position of feet, legs, and vertebral column when moving or walking.	Risk of fracture is increased if bones are markedly deformed or decalcified.
Listen to patient's concerns about possible fracture(s).	May be very reluctant to move because of weak bones.
Administer prescribed diet and discuss high-calcium foods and vitamin D foods.	Increased intake and utilization of calcium and vitamin D are the treatments for osteomalacia.
Discuss purposes of physical therapy program, if prescribed.	Exercises increase retention of calcium in bones.
Instruct patient/family regarding a safe home environment: no long, uncovered or loose cords and no small, loose rugs.	Loose cords or rugs may lead to falls and fractures. Twisting may fracture fragile, demineralized bones.
Teach patient/family the effects of calcium and vitamin D on the body and factors affecting absorption and utilization.	Calcium is vital for bone strength, with 99% of the body's calcium being retained in bones. Calcium and vitamin D are absorbed in the small intestine. Sunlight is necessary for vitamin D metabolites to be converted to usable vitamin D in the body. Exercises are vital to retain calcium in bones.
Teach patient symptoms of a fracture: inability to bear weight or use part normally, increase in pain or soreness, and swelling or discoloration.	Bone fracture is loss of bone integrity, and the type of fracture may vary according to the bone and severity of the fracture (see Table 1.3, page 19).

▶ NURSING DIAGNOSIS: *Acute Pain*

Related To skeletal deformities and muscular stretching or strain or impingement of nerves

Defining Characteristics

- Muscular weakness
- Persistent, aching skeletal pain
- Radiating pain in back or down legs

Patient Outcomes

The patient will

- experience relief of pain with medications.
- regain normal bone and muscle functions.

Nursing Interventions	Rationales
Assess sites, amount, type, nature, severity, and duration of pain.	Pain is usually dull and aching but may be sharp and burning if nerve is impinged. There may be some numbness and tingling also. Pain is usually persistent.
Ask patient about effects of measures he or she has used to relieve pain.	The patient may have utilized methods to relieve pain with inconsistent results.
Assist patient to a position of comfort; encourage to change position q2–3h.	Positioning lessens strain on weak or tired muscles, thereby easing discomfort and pain.
Administer prescribed analgesics.	Nonnarcotic analgesic medications may be used initially. Narcotics may be used if insufficient relief is obtained from nonnarcotic analgesics, only until bone strength and shape are regained.
Gently massage back several times daily.	Massage eases tired, painful muscles and joints. Massage must be gentle to prevent trauma to bones.
Encourage compliance with physical therapy regimen, proper diet, plus intake of calcium and vitamin D.	As bones regain mineralization and strength, deformities decrease and pain is relieved.

DISCHARGE PLANNING/CONTINUITY OF CARE

- Refer to home care agency for follow-up care as needed.
- Refer to physical therapist for home exercise regimen.
- Discuss medication regimen (nonnarcotic medications) for pain control.
- Refer to dietitian for dietary guidelines to prevent recurrence of disease.

REFERENCES

Hoare, K., & Donohoe, K. M. (1990). Osteomalacia. In K. L. McCance & S. E. Huether (Eds.), *Pathophysiology* (p. 1330). St. Louis: Mosby.

Kim, M. J., McFarland, G. K., & McLane, A. M. (1993). *Pocket guide to nursing diagnoses* (5th ed.). St. Louis: Mosby-Yearbook.

Mourad, L. A. (1991). *Orthopedic disorders.* St. Louis: Mosby-Yearbook.

Mourad, L. A., & Droste, M. M. (1993). *The nursing process in the care of adults with orthopaedic conditions.* Albany: Delmar.

Salmond, S. W., Mooney, N. E., & Verdisco, L. A. (1991). *Core curriculum for orthopaedic nursing* (2nd ed.). Pitman NJ: Janetti.

OSTEOPOROSIS

Osteoporosis is a condition of imbalance between bone formation and bone resorption, leading to a decrease in total bone mass in the body. Persons with osteoporosis have bones that are smaller than normal, causing them to be unable to bear normal weights.

ETIOLOGIES

- Aging
- Caucasian
- Female gender (eight times more common in women than men)
- Hormone losses or deficiencies
- Hormone use (oral contraceptives)
- Imbalance between functions of osteoblasts and osteoclasts
- Immobility
- Low calcium intake
- Medications (aluminum-containing antacids, steroids, caffeine, nicotine)
- Menopause
- Oophorectomy
- Rheumatoid arthritis
- Sedentary life style
- Trauma, minor or sudden

CLINICAL MANIFESTATIONS

- Abnormal thoracic vertebral curvature
- Atrophy of muscles
- Back pain with or without radiation down leg
- Contracture of joints
- Deformity of vertebra(e)
- Fractures of one or more bones (hip, radius, vertebra)
- Loss of height

CLINICAL/DIAGNOSTIC FINDINGS

- Decreased levels of serum alkaline phosphatase
- Elevated serum calcium levels
- Kyphosis
- Roentgenographic evidence of compression fracture of vertebra and relative bone losses
- Single and double photon absortiometry reveals osteoporosis

▶ NURSING DIAGNOSIS: *Impaired Physical Mobility*

Related To fracture of vertebra(e), hip, or radius

Defining Characteristics

- Inability to bear weight or use part normally
- Presence of fracture of vertebra, hip, or radius

Patient Outcomes

The patient will

- experience healing of the fracture.
- regain physical mobility without ambulatory aid.

Nursing Interventions	Rationales
Assess site of fracture: note circulation, edema, color, temperature and pain; note sensory changes, such as numbness and tingling; note capillary refill, if pertinent; note bruising or soreness; note position of fracture site: if femur/hip, may be externally rotated and shortened; if radius, may have visible deformity or shortening.	A fracture is a break in a bone that, in osteoporosis, may result from minor trauma (see fractures, pages 3–16).
Support the injury site in a position of comfort but do not move injured tissues on own.	Movement can cause additional trauma.
Apply ice packs to injured tissues.	Ice decreases venous congestion, thereby lessening edema; arterial circulation is also lessened, decreasing hemorrhage or bleeding into the site; ice also lessens pain.
Assist with diagnostic regimen, if ongoing.	Patient may have roentgen studies, blood work, or other diagnostic studies prior to receiving definitive treatment of the fracture.
If proposed, assist with application of a cast to the forearm if a radial fracture.	A cast is a commonly used treatment after a radial fracture (see casts, pages 29–36).
Complete admission procedures and prepare patient for surgical repair of hip fracture, if present.	If osteoporosis is pronounced of femoral neck, the head of the femur may be replaced with a prosthesis;

Nursing Interventions	Rationales
	hip nails may be used if sufficient bone stock is present; surgery is usually done as soon as the patient's condition is stable. (See pages 199–212 for postoperative care after hip surgery.)
If the patient has a compression fracture of the vertebra, apply a back support, if prescribed.	Compression fractures of the vertebrae may be treated with a back support or just bedrest with the bed flat.
Perform all nine neurovascular checks, if pertinent.	Neurovascular checks provide data of vital concern in patient care (see page 21).
Assist patient to ambulate with use of walker or crutches, as prescribed.	Ambulation aids the patient's recovery and exercise helps retain calcium in bones.
Perform wound care if incision is present.	Wound healing without infection aids physical mobility. Healing requires aseptic care.
Turn patient side to side q3–4h.	Turning facilitates circulation and prevents formation of decubiti as well as easing tired muscles.

▶ NURSING DIAGNOSIS: *High Risk for Injury (Fracture)*

Risk Factors

- Bones unable to bear normal weights
- Decreased bone mass in body

Patient Outcomes

The patient will

- experience no fractured bone(s).
- regain strength in bones after treatments.

Nursing Interventions	Rationales
Assess patient's posture and gait; note varus "planting" of feet when walking.	Data are vital to planning care. Normally, the angle between the femur into the acetabulum is 135°; with aging and osteoporosis, the angle decreases, leading to a more varus placing of feet when walking. The sharpness of the angle, plus the weakened bones, increases the risk of femoral neck fracture. The increased kyphosis can lead to compression fractures of vertebrae.
Determine amount, site, duration, persistence, and time of pain, if present.	Pain may be indicative of muscle or joint pain or pressure on a nerve due to kyphosis or hip angle change. Pain may also be one indication of a stress fracture.
Assist patient with use of cane or crutches, if prescribed.	Use of an ambulatory aid lessens weight bearing on a weak or injured joint and can lessen risk of fracture of bone.
Assist patient with range-of-motion (ROM) exercises.	Range-of-motion exercises help muscles and joints retain strength and help keep calcium in bones. Swimming is an excellent exercise that does not increase the risk of fractures.
Teach about foods high in calcium and vitamin D.	Calcium is needed to make or keep bones strong and correctly shaped. Vitamin D enhances calcium absorption in the intestine. Calcium intake daily should be 1500 mg and vitamin D intake should be 400 IU daily in postmenopausal persons.
Discuss stopping smoking or intake of alcohol.	Both nicotine and alcohol increase the development of osteoporosis by causing excessive calcium loss.

Nursing Interventions	Rationales
Reiterate physician's explanations about purposes of estrogen and phosphonate (etidronate) intake.	Intake of estrogen alone (in posthysterectomy) or estrogen-progestin combinations in women with intact uteri plus etidronate lessens bone resorption and may increase bone formation.

▶ NURSING DIAGNOSIS: *Impaired Gas Exchange*

Related To increased kyphosis

Defining Characteristics

- Atrophy of paravertebral muscles
- Increased kyphosis
- Limited ability for back extension
- Vertebral fracture causing pain

Patient Outcomes

The patient will

- experience no respiratory infection.
- regain satisfactory respiratory functions.

Nursing Interventions	Rationales
Assess respiratory rates and depths; assess breath sounds in all lobes of lungs.	Assessments determine the extent of patient's respiratory deficits.
Encourage deep-breathing exercises q3–4h.	Deep breathing enhances gas exchange and lessens chance of development of atelectasis.
Assess sites, severity, duration, and type(s) of pain.	The site(s) of pain may be in the upper lateral, middle, or lower lateral back depending on which vertebral segments are fractured. Pain may be acute and disabling and aching or burning and can be referred to the anterior or lateral intercostal regions. Pain can also be referred to the flank and hip areas and lumbosacral areas.

Nursing Interventions	Rationales
Administer nonnarcotic analgesic, if prescribed.	Nonnarcotic analgesics relieve pain without depressing respirations. Persons breathe deeper when they are pain free or do not fear having pain because of medication intake.
Assist with the injection of a local anesthetic into the spinous processes or interspinous spaces or facet areas, if done.	Use of a local anesthetic injection relieves the chronic pain episodes for varying periods.
Consult physical therapists for appropriate, safe exercises.	An exercise regimen must enhance respiratory functions without causing more injury to the patient.

DISCHARGE PLANNING/CONTINUITY OF CARE

- Refer to home care agency for follow-up care if surgery performed.
- Arrange for follow-up physician's visit.
- Arrange for physical therapy for home exercise regimen.
- Review purposes and side effects of medications; provide written guidelines.

REFERENCES

Avioli, L. V. (1992). Significance of osteoporosis: A growing national health care problem, *Orthopaedic Review. 21*(9), 1126–1129.

Cooper, C., & Melton, L. J. (1992). Vertebral fractures. How large is the silent epidemic. *British Medical Journal, 304*, 793.

Felson, D. T., Sloutskis, D., Anderson, J. J., Anthony, K. M., & Kiel, D. P. (1991). Thiazide diuretics and the risk of hip fracture. *Journal of American Medical Association, 265*(3), 370–373.

Heaney, R. P., Avioli, L. V., & Chestnut, C. H. III (1989). Osteoporotic bone fragility: Detection by ultrasound transmission velocity. *Journal of American Medical Association, 261*(2O), 2986–2990.

Itoi, E., Yamada, Y., Sakurai, M., Sato, K., & Kasama, F. (1992). Long-term treatment with 1-hydroxyvitamin D_3 with calcium supplement in spinal osteoporotic patients. *Orthopedics, 15*(12), 1409–1415.

Jenkins, E. A., & Cooper, C. (1993). The epidemiology of osteoporosis: Who is at risk? *Journal of Musculoskeletal Medicine, 10*(3) 18–33.

Kelly, E. J., Eisman, J. A., & Sambrook, P. W. (1990). Interaction of genetic and environmental influences on peak bone density. *Osteoporosis International, 1*(1), 56–60.

Kiel, D. R., Baron, J. A., Anderson, J. J., Hannan, M. T., & Felson, D. T. (1992). Smoking cancels protective effect of estrogen on bones. *Annals of Internal Medicine, 116*(5), 716–721.

Liscum, B. (1992). Osteoporosis: The silent disease. *Journal of Orthopaedic Nursing, 10*(4), 21–25.

Meyeroff, W., & Pope, T. (1993). WHO European study compares prophylactics for osteoporosis, *Orthopedics Today, 13*(3), 28.

Perloff, J. J., McDermott, M. T., Perloff, K. G., Blue, P. W., Enzenhauer, R., Sieck, E., Chantelois, A. E., Dolbow, A., & Kidd, G. S. (1991). Reduced bone-mineral content is a risk factor for hip fractures. *Orthopaedic Review, 20*(8), 689–698.

Salmond, S. W., Mooney, N. E., & Verdisco, L. A. (1991). *Core curriculum for orthopaedic nursing* (2nd ed.). Pitman NJ: Janetti.

Slemenda, C. W., Christian, J. C., Reed, T., Reister, T. K., Williams, C. J., & Johnston, C. C., Jr. (1992). Long-term bone loss in men: Effects of genetic and environmental factors. *Annals of Internal Medicine, 117,* 286–291.

Wilkes, L. L., & Barnhill, S. D. (1992). Biochemical measurement of bone mineral density: The significance of lymphocyte alkaline phosphatase isoenzyme. *Contemporary Orthopaedics, 25*(6), 580–584.

Wilkes, L. L., & Barnhill, S. D. (1992). Osteoporosis: An autoimmune disease. *Journal of Bone and Joint Surgery, 74-B*, 234.

GOUT AND GOUTY ARTHRITIS

Gout is a metabolic condition of a defect in purine metabolism leading to hyperuricemia. The excess urates are deposited in body tissues and joints.

Gouty arthritis is secondary to the deposit of monourate crystals in joint spaces. The crystals are deposited in joints and other body areas because of a buildup of uric acid. Uric acid builds up because of incomplete metabolism of purines from lack of the enzyme needed for complete purine metabolism, which is the disease called gout.

ETIOLOGIES

- Buildup of uric acid crystals in body due to incomplete metabolism of purines
- Increased production of uric acid secondary to increased cell destruction from medications given for malignant diseases, such as leukemia

CLINICAL MANIFESTATIONS

- Appearance of tophi
- Arthritic deformities of joints
- Exquisite pain in large toe or other joints
- Inflammation in affected joints

CLINICAL/DIAGNOSTIC FINDINGS

- Elevated serum uric acid
- Exquisitely painful, inflamed joints on palpation
- Joint fluid analysis shows characteristic urate crystals
- Presence of tophi in pinnae of ears and metacarpal joints

► NURSING DIAGNOSIS: *Acute Pain*

Related To build up and characteristics of urate crystals (sharp, pointed, needlelike) in joint tissues

Defining Characteristics

- Hot, inflamed joints
- Sudden, severe pain in joint(s), most commonly the first metatarso-phalangeal joint of great toe; other joints are wrist and metacarpal joints

Patient Outcomes

The patient will

- control gout with diet and medications.
- experience only mild pain during acute attacks of gouty arthritis.

Nursing Interventions	Rationales
Assess site(s), severity, duration, type, and persistence of pain.	During acute attacks of inflammatory gout, the patient will experience exquisite pain, described as "sharp needles sticking through my joints." The pain persists until treated with medications.
Place patient on bedrest during acute attack; keep covers off imflamed joint.	Bedrest lessens strain on acutely inflamed joint(s). Keeping covers off inflamed joints lessens pressure on them.
Apply ice bag to inflamed joint(s).	Ice constricts circulation and lessens edema and pain.
Administer prescribed medication, most commonly colchicine (colsalsid).	Colchicine is usually given in 1-mg doses orally initially, then 0.5 mg every hour until the patient experiences diarrhea or headache, signs of therapeutic levels. The pain is usually markedly relieved in six to eight doses. More than 8 mg in 8 h can reach toxic levels and should be avoided.
Administer allopurinol or probenecid, if prescribed.	These medications are given to prevent acute attacks, when possible, and are about 75% effective in doing so.
Monitor effects and side effects of medications.	Colchicine causes severe diarrhea and headache when given to toxic levels. Dosage during an acute attack is therefore limited to 8 mg.

Nursing Interventions	Rationales
Teach patient/family to control gout through diet.	Dietary intake of high-purine-containing foods (see Table 13.1, below) exacerbates attacks of gout. Recurrent attacks can be controlled by maintaining lower intake of purine-containing foods.
Teach patient about long-term control of gout through use of allopurinol or probenecid.	These medications must be taken daily to increase the excretion of uric acid to help prevent acute attacks of gout.

DISCHARGE PLANNING/CONTINUITY OF CARE

- Refer to dietitian for diet low in purines for home use.
- Discuss purposes and side effects of medications for home use.
- Arrange for follow-up physician's visit.

Table 13.1 • Purine Content of Foods

High (150-1,000 mg/100g)	Moderate (50-150 mg/100g)	Negligible
Herring	Chicken	Vegetable soups
Sardines	Crab	Butter
Mussels	Salmon	Refined cereals
Liver	Veal	Eggs
Sweetbreads	Mutton	Fruits
Kidney	Bacon	Vegetables
Venison	Pork	Cheese
Goose	Beef	Milk
Meat soups	Ham	Sugar
Anchovies	Lentils	
Brains	Whole-grain cereals	
Heart	Beans	
	Spinach	
	Asparagus	
	Cauliflower	

Source: From The nursing process in the care of adults with orthopaedic conditions, *3rd. ed., by Mourad, L. A. and Droste, M. M., 1993, Albany, NY: Delmar. Copyright 1993 by Delmar Publishers Inc. Reprinted by permission.*

REFERENCES

Dowd, S. B. (1993). The radiographic appearance of gout. *Journal of Orthopaedic Nursing, 12*(1), 53–56.

Fudman, E. J., & Fox, I. H. (1993). When clinical clues point to gout. *Journal of Musculoskeletal Medicine, 10*(2), 64–75.

Kim, M. J., McFarland, G. K., & McLane, A. M. (1993). *Pocket guide to nursing diagnoses* (5th ed.). St. Louis: Mosby-Yearbook.

Mourad, L. A. (1991). *Orthopedic disorders.* St. Louis: Mosby-Yearbook.

Mourad, L. A., & Droste, M. M. (1993). *The nursing process in the care of adults with orthopaedic conditions* (3rd ed.). Albany: Delmar.

PAGET'S DISEASE

Paget's disease, or osteitis deformans, is a skeletal disorder in which there is marked bone resorption with excessive localized overgrowth of bone. Bones become greatly deformed and unevenly remodeled, with structurally unsound bones. Areas commonly involved include the bones of the face, skull, jaws, long bones, and spine.

ETIOLOGIES

- Possibly, virus of paramyxoviridae family
- Unknown cause of imbalance between bone formation and resorption

CLINICAL MANIFESTATIONS

- Bone deformities
- Bone overgrowth
- Development of bowlegs
- Fatigue
- Increased skin temperature over affected bone(s)
- Intense skeletal pain
- Skull enlargement

CLINICAL/DIAGNOSTIC FINDINGS

- Elevated serum alkaline phosphatase
- Pathologic fracture
- Roentgenographs showing thickened bone cortex and deformed bones

NOTE: Nursing diagnoses of impaired physical mobility, high risk for injury (fracture), and acute pain and the associated outcomes and interventions are very similar to those discussed under osteomalacia and osteoporosis. The reader is directed to those areas to prevent repetition.

DISCHARGE PLANNING/CONTINUITY OF CARE

- Arrange for follow-up appointments for medical care and for physical or occupational therapy.
- Contact community health nurses through the continuity-of-care referral for assessment of physical health status, medication regime, and possible side effects of medications.

Clinical Clip

Osteoporosis leads to more than 1.3 million fractures in the United States alone, exceeding $10 billion in costs (MacDougall, 1991).

In the United States, about 2.6 persons per 1,000 have gouty arthritis.

REFERENCES

Hoare, K., & Donohoe, K. M. (1990). Paget disease. In K. L. McCance & S. E. Huether (Eds.), *Pathophysiology* (pp. 1331–1332). St. Louis: Mosby-Yearbook.

Kim, M. J., McFarland, G. K., & McLane, A. M. (1993). *Pocket guide to nursing diagnoses* (5th ed.). St. Louis: Mosby-Yearbook.

Louthrenoo, W., & Schumacher, H. R. (1990). Musculoskeletal clues to endocrine or metabolic disease. *Journal of Musculoskeletal Medicine, 7*(9), 33–58.

MacDougall, D.S. (1991). Meeting highlights: Third international symposium on osteoporosis. *Orthopaedic Review, 20*(3), 284–291.

Mourad, L. A. (1991). *Orthopedic disorders.* St. Louis: Mosby-Yearbook.

Salmond, S. W., Mooney, N. E., & Verdisco, L. A. (1991). *Core curriculum for orthopaedic nursing* (2nd ed.). Pitman NJ: Janetti.

Infections of Bones and Bone Marrow

Infections of bones, bone marrow, or joints can cause prolonged illness and are to be avoided when possible. Patients with open wounds, sore throat, or urinary tract or systemic infections are at increased risks for development of osteomyelitis. Children are prone to develop hematogenous or blood-borne infection, commonly caused by coagulase-positive *Staphylococcus aureus*. If the infectious organisms cross the epiphysis and the infection spreads, growth arrest can occur due to destruction of the growth plate.

OSTEOMYELITIS

Osteomyelitis is infection of bone and the bone marrow. It can result from direct invasion from an open wound or from indirect invasion secondary to infection in other parts of the body. It commonly develops when the person's resistance is low or when there is decreased flow of blood at the site of development of osteomyelitis. Also, persons with sickle cell disease get osteomyelitis from the lowered oxygen tension they experience. Inadequately treated acute osteomyelitis can go on to become chronic osteomyelitis.

ETIOLOGIES

- *Escherichia coli*
- *Neisseria gonorrhoeae*
- *Salmonella typhi*
- *Staphylococcus aureus*—causes nearly 90% of purulent osteomyelitis
- Streptococci
- Methicillin-resistant *Staphylococcus*

CLINICAL MANIFESTATIONS

- Fever, both systemic and local
- Pain and lack of desire to use affected limb
- Presence of infected area, most commonly in metaphyseal area of bone
- Presence of inflamed area in affected bone
- Purulent drainage through fistulous track
- Complaints of fatigue, weakness, headache, and nausea

CLINICAL/DIAGNOSTIC FINDINGS

- Culture of drainage revealing infecting organisms
- Elevated erythrocyte sedimentation rate
- Elevated white blood cells, with 80% polymorphonuclear neutrophils (normal is 50–70%)
- Fistulous track with purulent drainage
- History of open trauma or antecedent infection

- Inflamed area with redness, edema, and elevated skin temperature
- Radiographs may show bone destruction
- Systemic temperature elevation of 101–104 F (38.3–40 C)
- Teichoic acid antibody test may show antibodies

▶ NURSING DIAGNOSIS: *Impaired Physical Mobility*

Related To inflamed and infected bone

Defining Characteristics

- Inflamed or infected area in bone
- Reluctance to use part
- Systemic fever

Patient Outcomes

The patient will

- experience no recurrence of infection.
- regain physical mobility after treatments.

Nursing Interventions	Rationales
Assess site of inflammation; observe for drainage, mass, elevated skin temperature, and painful area.	Site may have incisional area if secondary to surgical intervention; may have fistulous track with odorous drainage; patient does not want anyone to touch area and does not want to move the affected limb.
Assist patient to a position of comfort.	If a limb is involved, it should be lifted at the joints above and below the inflamed area. It can also be placed on a pillow for more comfort.
Maintain bedrest, if prescribed.	Bedrest decreases fatigue and metabolic demands in a weakened host. The patient may be allowed bathroom privileges.
Demonstrate use of crutches, if to be used when ambulatory.	Proper technique for crutch use is a safety concern in a weakened person.

▶ NURSING DIAGNOSIS: *Ineffective Thermoregulation—Hyperthermia*

Related To infection and temperatures of 101–104 F (38.3–40 C)

Defining Characteristics

- Confusion or altered time perception
- Localized raised skin temperature in affected area
- Restlessness
- Spiking systemic temperatures and chills

Patient Outcomes

The patient will

- regain normal body temperatures after treatments.
- regain healing of infected area.

Nursing Interventions	Rationales
Assess vital signs and temperature as prescribed; report marked elevations to physician.	All vital signs are raised with hyperthermia. Blood pressure and pulse rates increase to get more oxygen into all cells; respirations increase to bring in more oxygen and aid excretion of waste carbon dioxide. The temperatures increase to help create an environment to kill the pathogen and in response to the pathogenic invasion in the body.
Assist with obtaining blood cultures, if prescribed.	Blood cultures may be drawn during hyperthermic periods to determine the pathogen if septicemia is present.
Administer prescribed antibiotics.	Antibiotics are given intravenously for up to 6 weeks followed by oral administration.
Administer aspirin or acetaminophen q4h, as prescribed.	Antipyretics such as aspirin or acetaminophen help lower high temperatures, which may affect neural structures and functions. **NOTE:** Aspirin should not be given to children or teens because of its association with Reye syndrome.

Nursing Interventions	Rationales
Change gown and bed linens if they become damp.	When fever drops, perspiration and diaphoresis occur, causing clothing and bed linens to become damp and cold.
If patient is a child and temperature remains above 102–104 F (38.8–40 C) for long periods, observe child for seizures or convulsions.	Children with high fevers are susceptible to convulsions and should be observed frequently in the event of such occurrence.
Offer fluids q1–2h; observe skin turgor and mucous membranes for moistness.	Diaphoresis increases insensible water losses which should be replaced with oral fluids.

▶ NURSING DIAGNOSIS: *Acute Pain*

Related To presence of mass, infection, and altered tissue perfusion

Defining Characteristics

- Complaints of severe pain at site of infection
- Guarding or protective behavior of affected limb
- Moaning or crying
- Restlessness

Patient Outcomes

The patient will

- have a decrease or relief of pain.
- have normal tissue perfusion.
- reuse the affected limb without discomfort.

Nursing Interventions	Rationales
Assess degree, intensity, duration, and type of pain.	Pain is due to the pressure of the mass on nerve endings. The pain is usually intense, constant, and aching.
Assist patient to adjust positions for comfort; handle affected limb gently.	A person in pain is restless and has difficulty finding or holding a comfortable position. Always handle a tender or sore limb under the joints above and below the affected area.

Nursing Interventions	Rationales
Administer analgesics as prescribed.	Until the infection is relieved, analgesics help relieve the pain episodes.
Provide games, cards, puzzles, and other supplies for diversion.	Diversionary activities divert the person's attention from the pain and help the passage of time.
Do neurovascular checks as prescribed; compare with opposite limb for patient's parameters.	See page 21 for all neurovascular checks.
Accompany patient to hyperbaric therapy department, if necessary, to aid in transferring patient to chamber.	Hyperbaric oxygen therapy may be used for increasing the oxygen perfusion to the bone. The patient must be placed in the hyperbaric chamber. Moving may be painful, and having a trusted person move the affected limb lessens the patient's concerns.

▶ NURSING DIAGNOSIS: *Impaired Skin Integrity*

Related To the presence of purulent drainage, irrigation tubes, and osteomyelitis

Defining Characteristics

- Fistulous track from internal osteomyelitis to skin
- Open, draining wound
- Presence of an external fixator
- Tubes inserted into osteomyelitis site

Patient Outcomes

The patient will

- experience no recurrence of osteomyelitis.
- regain an intact skin area after treatments.

Nursing Interventions	Rationales
Assess infection site for type and amount of drainage.	Drainage may be greenish in color, have a pungent odor, and be profuse.

Nursing Interventions	Rationales
Assess drainage from irrigating tubes.	Irrigating tubes may be inserted into the site of osteomyelitis after surgery to remove sequestrum (dead bone). Antibiotics in solution are flushed through the tubes and fluid is then removed. The antibiotics clear the infection from the site.
Check the pins, nuts, and bolts of the external fixator every shift.	The external fixator may be placed with pins (rods) above and below the infected area to prevent a pathologic fracture.
Use strict aseptic technique for wound care and dressing changes; dispose of dressings using universal precautions.	Aseptic technique prevents introduction of organisms into the area and prevents transfer of infection to others.
Perform pin care to pins of external fixator, if institutional policy.	Pin care may consist of cleansing the entrance and exit sites with hydrogen peroxide and sterile saline, drying the sites, then covering with small dressings of sterile Kerlex (expandable cotton dressing). Pin care may not be done if the pin sites are clean, dry, noninflamed, or drainage free.
Observe wound site for healing or continuing drainage or infection.	Wound sites may be small and closed with skin clips or sutures or may be extensive, requiring a skin graft for closure. Healing is noted by lack of warmth, redness, edema, draining, or pain, with skin surfaces closed and intact.

▶ NURSING DIAGNOSIS: *Knowledge Deficit*

Related To suddenness or newness of diagnosis or treatments

Defining Characteristics

- Antecedent infection approximately 10 days to 2 weeks previously that has resolved
- Open wound with foreign substances including dirt

- Treatment regimen to include intravenous antibiotics, surgical saucerization, hyperbaric oxygen therapy, and irrigating tubes

Patient Outcomes

The patient will
- participate actively in the decisions regarding his or her treatments.
- understand the purposes of proposed treatments and their effects.

Nursing Interventions	Rationales
Assess patient's knowledge of meaning of osteomyelitis, the treatments, and their effects.	Determining the patient's understandings is the basis for further teaching.
Clarify the physician's explanations; listen to patient's concerns.	Clarifying and listening help patient regain or gain a sense of worth and power.
Use appropriate words, pictures, or diagrams to help clarify treatments.	Patient's ways of learning vary, and different methods enhance learning.
Encourage patient to participate in decisions regarding the treatment regimen.	Active participation helps the patient cope with the healing process and treatments.
Keep the patient informed of upcoming treatments as needed.	Being aware of progress and plans helps patient participate actively and positively.
Provide diversionary activities.	Having activities to divert attention prevents patient from unhealthy self-absorption.

DISCHARGE PLANNING/CONTINUITY OF CARE

- Teach self-care, including care of a wound/incision, self-administration of antibiotics and analgesics, and possible use of ambulatory aids, if needed.
- Complete continuity-of-care referral for assessment of self-care at home.

REFERENCES

Almekinders, L. C., & Lachiewicz, P. F. (1991). Nocardia osteomyelitis. *Orthopedics, 12*(12), 1583–1585.

Hackford, A. W. (1992). Orthopedic manifestations of retroperitoneal infection. *Complications in Orthopedics, 7*(4), 262–266.

Heyne, C. (1992). Wound care in the elderly. *Reflections, 18*(4), 8.

Hoekman, P., Van de Perre, P., & Nelissen, J. (1991). Increased frequency of infection after open reduction of fractures in patients who are seropositive for human immunodeficiency virus. *Journal of Bone and Joint Surgery, 73A*(5), 675–679.

Kelman, G. J., Roland, G. C., & Beagley, M. J. (1993). Acute *Pseudomonas* infection following total hip replacement. *Orthopedics, 16*(2), 209–214.

Kieser, L. (1992). Complications of knee surgery. *Arthroscopy, 8*(1), 82.

Martin, M. E. (1989). Oral antibiotics for treatment of patients with chronic osteomyelitis. *Journal of Orthopaedic Nursing, 8*(3), 35–38.

Schmalzried, T. P., Amstutz, H. C., Au, M., & Dorey, F. J. (1991). Incidence of deep sepsis in total hip arthroplasty. *Journal of Arthroplasty, 6*(Suppl.), S47–S51.

Schurman, D. J. (moderator), Esterhai, J. L., Gristina, A. G., Lidgren, L., & Nelson, C. L. (1992). Symposium: Infection control in orthopaedics. *Contemporary Orthopaedics, 25*(6), 609–626.

Thoren, B., & Wigren, A. (1991). Erythrocyte sedimentation rate in infection of total hip replacements. *Orthopedics, 14*(4), 495–497.

Musculoskeletal Tumors

Bone tumors are either benign or malignant and account for about 3% of all malignant tumors. Malignant bone tumors affect children, teenagers, and young adults most frequently and account for less than 1% of all deaths from cancer. Most bone tumors are primary, but secondary tumors occur as metastatic tumors. The most common malignant bone tumor is osteosarcoma (See Table 16.1, page 164, for listing of benign and malignant musculoskeletal tumors, their diagnostic procedures, and the usual treatments.)

OSTEOSARCOMA

Osteosarcoma accounts for about 35% of all malignant bone tumors. It is highly malignant, with rapid, agressive growth. Its peak incidence is between ages 10 and 20 and occurs slightly more often in males than in females.

ETIOLOGIES

- None known: associated with Paget's disease in persons between ages 50 and 60

CLINICAL MANIFESTATIONS

- Dull, aching, constant pain, often worse at night
- Mass in distal femur, proximal tibia, humerus, or mandible
- Reluctance to use affected part

CLINICAL/DIAGNOSTIC FINDINGS

- Bone scan shows "hot spot" at tumor site.
- Chest roentgenogram may show metastases, if present.
- Elevated serum alkaline phosphatase.
- Site roentgenograms show characteristic "sunburst" appearance.

▶ NURSING DIAGNOSIS: *Impaired Physical Mobility*

Related To tumor mass and pressure

Defining Characteristics

- Enlarging mass at tumor site, usually distal femur or proximal tibia
- Feelings of tightness and pressure at tumor site
- Reluctance to use affected part

Patient Outcomes

The patient will

- have relief of pressure after treatments.
- regain satisfactory mobility with treatments.

Nursing Interventions	Rationales
Assess site for presence of mass, skin tightness, and complaints of pressure.	These data are indications of size of tumor mass.
Place patient in positions of comfort; use pillows, if needed.	Positioning may be difficult because of size of tumor. Elevating on a pillow may lessen pressure symptoms.
Prepare patient for diagnostic tests which may include computerized tomography (CT) scan, bone scan, magnetic resource imaging (MRI), or x-ray; blood studies include complete blood count, alkaline or acid phosphatase, and others.	Diagnosis of specific types of bone tumors is difficult and often requires multiple diagnostic studies.
Assist patient to ambulate with cane or crutches, if prescribed.	An ambulatory aid may ease soreness and pressure plus prevent a possible pathologic fracture.
Assist with range-of-motion (ROM) exercises; use caution with joints near tumor site.	Range-of-motion exercises help maintain strength in unaffected muscles and joints.
If surgery is performed, reposition patient q2–3h.	Repositioning aids circulation, eases tired muscles, and hastens recovery as well as prevents complications.
Maintain the desired position of operative limb if limb salvage surgery done; position prescribed may be neutral, abducted, adducted, or internally or externally rotated. The foot of the bed may be elevated.	Desired position is dependent upon type of limb salvage surgery done. Elevation lessens edema formation by increasing venous return.
Consult physical therapist to assist with ambulation if hemipelvectomy or amputation is done of lower limb.	Patient may be "unbalanced" because of medications or loss of body part.
Assist orthotist with measuring for postoperative prosthesis, if prescribed and necessary.	Various types of prostheses are available, but exact fitting is needed for safe use.
Position patient for postoperative stretching exercises to prevent contractures: may do adduction or extension exercises.	Such exercises prevent the development of flexion contractures.

▶ NURSING DIAGNOSIS: *Acute Pain*

Related To enlarging mass, pressure on nerves, or other tissues (incision site)

Defining Characteristics

- Dull, aching constant pain, often worse at night
- Mass in bone, enlarging over time
- Presence of incisional area after surgery

Patient Outcomes

The patient will

- experience pain relief after medications and surgery.
- have no incisional pain after wound healing.

Nursing Interventions	Rationales
Assess type, amount, duration, and site of pain.	These data determine need for pain relief behaviors.
Reposition patient q2–3h.	Changing positions ease painful, tired muscles and joints.
During diagnostic regime, monitor for deformity, inability to bear weight, or sudden increase in pain.	These data may be indicative of a pathologic fracture.
Observe patient for sleeplessness, restlessness, wincing, crying, or withdrawal.	These are all signs of discomfort or pain.
Administer prescribed analgesic; after surgery, patient may use patient-controlled analgesia (PCA) pump to administer own analgesic; monitor use of PCA pump and relief of pain.	Analgesic medications may be nonnarcotic, anti-inflammatory, narcotic analgesics, or combinations of these. The PCA pump contains small amounts of narcotics per milliliter for more frequent self-administration.
Use splint, pillows, or immobilizer to position limb.	These appliances help the patient maintain a desirable position.
Massage back and tired muscles several times a day; assist with ROM exercises q4h.	Massage increases circulation to rid body of pain-producing wastes; ROM exercises ease tired or sore muscles to lessen pain.

Nursing Interventions	Rationales
Teach relaxation techniques, if appropriate.	These techniques help the patient regain control and power as well as ease pain.
Respond promptly to patient's complaints of pain if PCA pump not present.	Dealing promptly with the patient's concerns builds trust, lessens anxiety, and increases comfort.

▶ NURSING DIAGNOSIS: *Impaired Integumentary Tissue Perfusion*

Related To enlarging tumor

Defining Characteristics

- Edema distal to enlarging mass
- Enlarging mass in extremity
- Tight, taut shiny skin over enlarging mass

Patient Outcomes

The patient will

- have removal of enlarging mass.
- regain adequate peripheral tissue perfusion.
- regain intact integumentary tissues.

Nursing Interventions	Rationales
Assess neurovascular status of affected tissues.	These checks give data of degree or severity of impairment of perfusion (see neurovascular checks, page 21).
When moving the affected extremity, support the limb under the joints above and below.	Supporting at the joints helps maintain the strength of the limb and does not increase pain.
Elevate affected extremity on pillows; apply ice compress if desired.	Elevation helps increase venous return and lessen edema. Ice constricts vessels to lessen edema.
Monitor skin tissues to note any breaks or color changes.	The enlarging mass may stretch skin tissues so severely that the cells separate from each other; color may be white if tightly stretched.

Nursing Interventions	Rationales
Perform Homan sign by dorsiflexing patient's foot.	Homan sign is considered positive if the patient feels pain deep in the calf of the leg; it is an indication of phlebitis.

▶ NURSING DIAGNOSIS: *High Risk for Infection*

Risk Factors

- Decreased immunity due to chemotherapy
- Insertion of metallic devices

Patient Outcomes

The patient will

- experience no wound infection.
- have removal of skin clips without wound separation.
- regain intact skin with a well-healed scar.

Nursing Interventions	Rationales
Assess incisional area for presence of dressing, drainage tubes (Hemovac), and type and amount of drainage.	Presence of an incisional area removes the body's first line of defense against infection, thus predisposing the patient to a high risk of infection.
Monitor vital signs as prescribed; record and report elevation in temperature if over 101 F (38.4 C) and tachycardia above 100–110.	Elevated temperatures and tachycardia are two signs of systemic infection.
Check patient's chart to learn of presence of internal fixation devices, bone grafts, or catheters.	Metallic, plastic, cadaveric, or autologous bone implants or rubber catheters inside the body increase the risk of infection.
If external fixator is present, check all pin sites for presence, type, and amount of drainage.	A small amount of serosanguineous drainage around the pin sites is normal for 1–3 days after insertion, after which the sites are usually dry.
Perform "pin site care" according to physician or institution policy.	Such care may consist of inspecting the pin sites, cleansing away

Nursing Interventions	Rationales
	drainage with half-strength hydrogen peroxide/saline solution, drying the sites, and wrapping sites with small amounts of stretch gauze (Kerlex), and doing care every 3 days only if sites are not infected.
Change dressings at incision site using strict aseptic technique.	Strict asepsis lessens risk of infection transmission.
Identify agents which add to risk of infection, such as presence of intravenous catheters, needles, and tubing; chemotherapy; or radiation therapy.	Intravenous catheters, needles, or tubing may allow pathogens to enter and multiply, increasing chances of infection. Chemotherapy and radiation therapy reduce the number of white blood cells, predisposing to infection.
Review all medications which may mask infection.	Medications such as corticosteroids, phenylbutazone, antibiotics, antipyretics, and others may mask presence of infection.
Discuss factors of or conditions which increase the risk of infection to the patient.	Being in the hospital, changes in levels of immunoglobulin, presence of histocompatibility antigens, and others alter the patient's immune responses and increase the risk of infection.
Monitor all orifices for amount, type, and character of drainage.	Increases and changes in any of these parameters may signify presence of infection in one or more areas.
Monitor wound for signs of inflammation/infection: changes in color (redness), edema, increased heat in area, change in drainage from clear to cloudy to purulent, increased tenderness or soreness in area around wound (cellulitis), sore throat, urinary urgency, and such.	These changes are related to inflammation or infection, bringing increased blood to the area, increased metabolism in the area, increased debris and wastes in the area, capillary fragility and vasodilation, and local walling off of site by phagocytic white blood cells.
Monitor changes in systemic signs of infection: increased white blood cell (WBC) counts, chills and fever,	Total WBC counts increase in bacterial infections, with changes in cell differential counts; total WBC

Nursing Interventions	Rationales
malaise, redness or rash, diaphoresis, headache, low back pain, and others.	counts decrease in viral infections, with changes also in cell differential counts. The remaining patterns listed are systemic efforts to overcome pathogens in the body.
Use medical aseptic techniques and precautions to prevent nosocomial infections.	Persons with decreased resistance, which increases the host's susceptibility, are very prone to infections. Medical asepsis is a way to lessen the risks of nosocomial infection.

▶ NURSING DIAGNOSIS: *Body Image Disturbance*

Related To loss of a body part (amputation), large prominent scar, resection with limb-sparing surgery, or other repair

Defining Characteristics

- Absence of upper or lower extremity
- Postoperative condition after forequarter amputation, hemipelvectomy, rotationoplasty, or other surgery to resect and remove tumor
- Presence of stump after above-knee amputation

Patient Outcomes

The patient will

- express acceptance of altered body image.
- learn self-care as needed.
- regain a positive body image over time.

Nursing Interventions	Rationales
Assess person's concerns, as appropriate.	Initially postoperatively the person may need all energy for physical recovery and not be able to verbalize body image concerns.
Provide time and environment for patient to verbalize concerns when ready.	Trust must be built up over time for patient to discuss concerns with health care professionals.
Listen to patient's expressions of impact of changes on self, family,	Listening is an effective communication means for staff to develop

Nursing Interventions	Rationales
employment, activities of daily living (ADL), or other activities.	strategies to help patient regain independence.
Assist patient to participate in self-care such as use of walker or crutches to ambulate and adjustments in ADL as needed.	Assistance while practicing with unfamiliar equipment gives support and comfort to the patient.
Teach patient wound and dressing techniques as necessary.	Learning self-care helps the patient regain confidence and feel more positive about self.
Encourage patient to participate in support group activities, if appropriate.	Learning of others' experiences, if similar to patient's, helps patient feel less isolated or alone and is generally very beneficial.
Arrange for orthotist for measuring and fitting of prosthesis when wound healing is sufficient for weight bearing.	Proper measurement and fitting of prosthesis help the patient develop a more positive body image.

▶ NURSING DIAGNOSIS: *Altered Role Performance*

Related To amputation

Defining Characteristics

- Amputation of upper or lower extremity
- Resection of malignant tumor from limb

Patient Outcomes

The patient will

- regain satisfactory roles after wound healing and treatments.
- return to majority of roles using prosthesis.

Nursing Interventions	Rationales
Assess restrictions on patient's movements and activities due to amputation.	Restrictions vary whether it is an upper or lower extremity amputation or a forequarter (entire upper extremity) or hemipelvectomy (entire lower extremity and hip joint).

Nursing Interventions	Rationales
Monitor patient's abilities to ambulate with walker or crutches if lower extremity.	Patient may feel "unbalanced" following loss of limb.
Assist patient to use walker or crutches, as needed.	The patient may need help to maintain balance until strength returns and techniques are learned.
Assist patient with active (or passive) ROM exercises to unaffected joints; seek consultation with physical therapist as needed.	Range-of-motion exercises help maintain strength in musculoskeletal tissues and prevent atrophy and weakness. Active exercises are more strengthening than passive ones. Physical therapists use repetitive and resistive programs for more effective results for patients.
Confer with and coordinate efforts of health team members including social workers, physical and occupational therapist, orthotist, medical oncologist or radiation therapist, dietitian, and pharmacist.	Persons with specialized services should be utilized to help the patient regain health and return to usual roles.
Teach patient side effects of medications and discuss chemotherapy regimen, if being undertaken.	A combination of chemotherapeutic agents may be given for malignant bone tumors. All these agents have multiple side effects.
Provide information in written form. Provide written self-care procedures for home use.	Written instructions help assure that the patient has correct and sufficient information when at home.
Complete a continuity-of-care referral.	Care from community health nurses helps maintain recovery and provides the continuity until the patient regains a healthier state.

▶ NURSING DIAGNOSIS: *Altered Self-Concept*

Related To surgical ablation of tumor, presence of external fixator, and loss of hair after chemotherapy

Defining Characteristics

- Resection of osteosarcoma

- Loss of body parts (muscles, bone, skin, associated blood vessels) and functions of those parts
- Morbidity from extensive surgical resection, pre- and postoperative chemotherapy
- Loss of independence due to prolonged morbidity

Patient Outcomes

The patient will

- begin to regain a new self-concept over time.
- begin regaining self-identity and independence as recovery proceeds.
- tolerate chemotherapy regimen without undue side effects, except hair loss.

Nursing Interventions	Rationales
Assess reactions or responses to surgical resection and diagnosis.	Reactions may include grief and sadness over losses, regression to dependent behaviors, decreased attention to personal hygiene, decreased alertness, sleepiness and fatigue, and lack of interest in future.
Assess possible influences of medications.	Medications may cause some drowsiness, sleepiness, withdrawal, nausea, vomiting, or anorexia depending on frequency and dosage. Medications may be narcotics, nonnarcotic analgesics, muscle relaxants, antiemetics, chemotherapeutic drugs, or others.
Discuss patient's usual response to stressors.	Usual responses to stressors depend on the patient's perception of the threat and include the "fight-or-flight" behaviors of anger, hostility, aggressive or active participation in care, withdrawal, and excessive dependence. Behaviors vary with the age and maturity of the patient.
Include family members in discussions and care, as able.	If patient is young child, one or both parents may "speak" and act for child. Teenagers and young adults are just developing own

Nursing Interventions	Rationales
	independence and identities and require care givers' knowledge and skills to deal with their fluctuations in behaviors.
Assist patient/family members to set realistic goals.	Goals help patient/family members and health team plan and provide or assist with treatment regimen.
Allow open expression of feelings and concerns.	Expressions should be accepted as stated to help maintain a trusting atmosphere.
Determine effects of significant others' responses on patient.	Patient may take cues from responses of parents, siblings, friends, schoolmates, religious persons, and others and act from cues.
Use positive responses and behaviors of significant others to support patient during grief or morbidity from surgery or chemotherapy.	Positive actions help patient regain sense of control.
Discuss realistic, yet optimistic outcomes of condition and treatments.	Hearing of potential positive outcomes helps patient accept present state or reactions.
Discuss ways patient can regain independence and control while recovering from treatments.	Participation in self-care and learning helps patient regain control and independence.
Coordinate the various treatment regimens with appropriate personnel.	Coordination should lessen delays or double scheduling to help patient receive maximal benefits from treatments.
Encourage use of ambulatory aids as appropriate.	Aids may include use of crutches, wheelchair, or wagon, which increase patient's independence.
Secure physical or occupational therapy consultations as needed.	Special exercises or developmental/self-care skills may be required for child or teenager to regain independence or identity.
Offer praise and encouragement while patient practices skills or does self-care.	Learning and adjusting to needed changes takes practice and time and varies with each individual patient.

Nursing Interventions	Rationales
Provide baseball caps, turbans, scarves, or other items to cover bald head, as desired by patient.	Covering baldness from chemotherapy drugs lessens obvious differences of patient from peers and significant others.

▶ NURSING DIAGNOSIS: *Knowledge Deficit*

Related To newness of diagnosis of malignant tumor, diagnostic regimen, and proposed treatments

Defining Characteristics

- Multiple diagnostic tests, including blood studies, CT scan, chest x-ray MRI, and biopsy
- Possible diagnosis of osteosarcoma
- Potential upcoming limb salvage surgery or amputation

Patient Outcomes

The patient will

- develop full understanding of meaning of osteosarcoma and diagnostic and treatment regimen.
- participate actively in proposed plan of care.

Nursing Interventions	Rationales
Assess patient's/family's knowledge of potential diagnosis and plan of care.	Data provide basis for individualized care.
Gather information, charts, and diagrams to use in teaching plan.	Multiple aids are available for teaching patient/family.
Provide a private, quiet environment for teaching session.	Anxiety can interfere with learning. Learning about the patient's "specifics" is a private, family circumstance.
Clarify physician's explanations to date.	The proposed diagnostic/treatment regimen may not be able to be considered initially but may depend upon the patient's condition and readiness to learn.

Nursing Interventions	Rationales
Discuss proposed diagnostic and treatment regimens; use simple terms, charts, pictures, or diagrams to clarify presentation.	Because of newness and seriousness of potential diagnosis, a patient may need repetitive learning sessions to acquire a sound understanding. Patients learn best through a variety of methods.
Clarify unclear points as needed.	Patients may ask questions over several days or time periods to be sure of knowledge.
Repeat instructions for specific diagnostic procedures just prior to the examination.	Immediate need to know is a prime motivation to learn.
Review pre- and postoperative care according to proposed surgery.	Specific procedures are done depending on type of surgery. (See Table 16.1, page 162.)

NOTE: Nursing care of persons having muscle, cartilage, or fat tumors is similar to that given for bone tumors and will not be repeated to avoid redundancy. See Table 16.1 for types of tumor, diagnostic regimen, and usual treatments.

DISCHARGE PLANNING/CONTINUITY OF CARE

- Prepare written self-care instructions regarding stump wrapping, skin care, side effects of medications, going up and down stairs with crutches, application of a prosthesis, or other special care according to specific tumor and surgical resection.
- Contact community health nurses regarding the patient/family needs.
- Provide written lists of medications, dosages, and side effects; review carefully with patient and family.
- Consult with social workers for needed supplies or assistance with ongoing financial needs.

Clinical Clip

The most common malignant bone tumor is osteosarcoma.

Table 16.1 • Specific Characteristics, Diagnostic Procedures, and Usual Treatments for Bone and Muscle Tumors

Type of Tumor	Characteristics	Diagnostic Procedures	Usual Treatment
Tumors of bone			
Osteoma	Benign	Physical examination for site and size; bone scan may show increased uptake of radioisotope	Excision for relief of symptoms if needed; may be left untouched
Osteochondroma	Benign	X-ray or CT scan shows outpouching of trabecular bone at metaphyseal area of bone	Excision of tumor and resection of tendon to above its point of attachment to prevent recurrence (removes all precartilaginous connective tissues)
Chondroma or enchondroma	About 75% are benign; about 25% are malignant	X-ray or CT scan shows thinned bone cortex	En bloc wide excision if malignant; if malignant and in large long bone, amputation may be required
Chondroblastoma	Benign	X-ray or CT scan shows osteolytic lesion with dots or points of calcification	Excision with curettage and packing with bone chips; about one-third of these tumors recur
Giant cell tumor (osteoclastoma)	Benign	X-ray or CT scan shows bone-destroying (osteolytic) lesion with large, multilobular cells often resembling soap bubbles; radioisotope scan shows increased uptake	Careful, thorough excision in attempt to remove all tumor (has strong predilection for recurrence); if recurs, wide excision with bone grafts into defect is done; may be followed by radiation therapy
Giant cell tumor (osteoclastoma)	Malignant	X-ray, CT scan, or MRI study	En bloc wide excision with bone grafts or allograft if near joint; may amputate if there are repeated recurrences with malignant transformation

Table 16.1 • *continued*

Type of Tumor	Characteristics	Diagnostic Procedures	Usual Treatment
Aneurysmal bone cyst	Benign	X-rays show cystic lesion; arteriogram should demonstrate aneurysmic nature of cyst; MRI shows data similar to arteriograms	Curettage plus phenol to destroy bed or with cryosurgery (liquid nitrogen); radiation therapy is used only for inoperable lesions but is not used in areas of active cartilage growth
Unicameral bone cyst	Benign	X-rays show multiloculated cyst	Excision with bone grafts to defect; steroid injection into cyst; can recur
Osteosarcoma	Malignant	X-rays, CT scan, or MRI study show "sunburst" appearance characteristic of this tumor; may do tomogram x-rays; radionuclide scan helps determine tumor size and possible metastases, as does chest x-ray; serum alkaline phosphatase is elevated; arteriogram shows vascularity of tumor plus its relationship to contiguous tissues	Limb salvage with wide excision of tumor and surrounding tissues; may need joint replacement; excision of pulmonary metastatic lesions; both preoperative and postoperative chemotherapy and radiation therapy are also used; at times, limb amputation may be done
Parosteal osteosarcoma	Malignant, low grade	X-ray or CT scan shows tumor in metaphyseal area firmly attached to cortex of bone but nearly totally outside of bone (hence name of tumor); radionuclide scan shows increased uptake in tumor	Excision of tumor

Table 16.1 • *continued*

Type of Tumor	Characteristics	Diagnostic Procedures	Usual Treatment
Ewing's sarcoma	Malignant	X-ray, CT scan, or MRI study greatly aid diagnosis	Radiation therapy used, since tumor is radiosensitive; chemotherapy also used
Fibro-sarcoma	Malignant	X-ray, CT scan, or MRI study should outline lesion; may be in bone or soft tissues	En bloc wide excision
Tumors of Muscles			
Leiomyoma	Benign	Ultrasound studies of tumor mass (tumor develops in smooth muscle, commonly the uterus)	Surgical removal
Rhabdomy-oma	Benign	Physical examination of mass in skeletal (striated) muscle	Surgical removal
Leiomyo-sarcoma	Malignant	Ultrasound (smooth muscle tumor)	Removal with wide resection
Rhabdomy-osarcoma	Malignant	Arteriogram	Radiation therapy (tumor is radio-sensitive); surgical excision; chemo-therapy may be used

Source: From Orthopedic Disorders *by L. Mourad, 1991, St. Louis, MO: Mosby-Yearbook. Copyright 1991 by C. V. Mosby. Used by permission.*

REFERENCES

Grauer, P. (1993). Tools of the trade. *Education, Ohio Cancer Pain Initiative, 1*(1), 3.

Gulanick, M., Klopp, A., & Galanes, S. (1986). *Nursing care plans.* St. Louis: Mosby.

Kim, M. J., McFarland, G. K., & McLane, A. M. (1993). *Pocket guide to nursing diagnoses* (5th ed.). St. Louis, Mosby-Yearbook.

Mauer-Baack, C. (1993). Invited opinion. *Educator, Ohio Cancer Pain Initiative, 1*(1), 2.

Mourad, L. A. (1991). *Orthopedic disorders.* St. Louis: Mosby-Yearbook.

BONE MARROW TUMORS

Multiple myeloma, or plasma cell myeloma, is a malignant tumor of plasma cells in bone marrow. It causes destructive (osteolytic) lesions in bones throughout the body.

ETIOLOGIES

Possibilities include

- chronic hypersensitivity reactions?
- chronic inflammation?
- no determination of definite etiology.
- viral influences?

CLINICAL MANIFESTATIONS

- Insidious onset
- Loss of bone integrity, replaced by plasma cell tumors
- Pathologic fractures due to presence of tumors
- Severe pain in pelvis, spine, and ribs or other sites

CLINICAL/DIAGNOSTIC FINDINGS

- High concentration of serum immunoglobulin, specifically m-type immunoglobulin (Bence Jones protein)
- Anemia
- Anorexia
- Bone destruction by plasma cell tumors
- Confusion
- Granulocytopenia
- Hypercalcemia due to bone destruction
- Hyperuricemia due to increased cell destruction
- Activation of osteoclasts with increased bone resorption leading to osteoporosis
- Abnormally high levels of immunoglobulin G and occasionally IgA
- Polyuria: presence of Bence Jones protein, an abnormal globulin
- Thrombocytopenia

► NURSING DIAGNOSIS: *High Risk for Injury (Pathologic Fractures)*

Risk Factors

- Osteolytic tumors in many bones
- Tumor-weakened bones unable to bear normal weights

Patient Outcomes

The patient will

- experience no fractures or only stress fractures.
- receive treatments (chemotherapy) to lessen chance of fractures by destroying tumors.

Nursing Interventions	Rationales
Assess sites of skeletal pain; check x-ray findings to determine condition of bones.	These data help the nurse provide careful care.
Handle bones at two joints if moving patient in bed.	Handling at joints provides most support to weakened bones.
Assist the patient to ambulate, if allowed up.	Ambulation and exercise help calcium stay in bones or return to bones.
Provide a special bed, mattress, pillows, or supports.	Special beds and supports lessen risk of fractures.
Assist with administration of chemotherapeutic drugs.	Chemotherapeutic drugs are given to decrease the amount of plasma cells. Corticosteroid medications are also given for their antitumor effects.
If part of the therapeutic regimen, prepare the patient for radiation therapy.	Radiation therapy is given at specific sites for its palliative effects on these localized sites.
Administer other drugs as prescribed.	Allopurinol may be given to decrease serum uric acid levels. Furosemide may be given, along with intravenous saline, to increase renal excretion of calcium.
Consult physical therapists for a safe regimen of ambulation and range-of-motion (ROM) exercises.	Exercises and ambulation must be done carefully to lessen possibility of fractures.

▶ NURSING DIAGNOSIS: *Acute Pain*

Related To lesions (plasma cell tumors) in pelvis, spinal segments, ribs, and other bones

Defining Characteristics

- Osteolytic lesions in many bones
- Severe pain in one or more skeletal segments as given above

Patient Outcomes

The patient will

- experience control of pain with medications and localized radiation therapy.
- experience no untoward side effects from medications or radiation.

Nursing Interventions	Rationales
Assess sites, type, duration, characteristics, and amount of pain. Use pain scale (0–10, 10 being worst) for patient to communicate severity of pain.	Pain in multiple myeloma may be quite severe at one or more sites related to tumor masses. Use of a pain scale helps all persons involved communicate on similar levels.
Gently reposition patient q2–3h.	Repositioning eases tired, aching muscles and joints.
Gently massage back several times daily.	Massage eases muscle soreness, tenderness, and pain.
Administer nonnarcotic and/or narcotic analgesics, as prescribed, around the clock.	Initially, patients may have pain relief with acetaminophen and later acetaminophen with codeine may be given around the clock.
Apply back support or brace, if prescribed.	A support or brace helps relieve pain.
Monitor skin tissues being irradiated for local bone lesions.	Skin tissues receive radiation in the specific areas. Usually, no soaps, ointments (except vitamin A&D Ointment), or alcohol is to be used on these areas within the purple lined areas. Skin surfaces should be checked for color changes, presence of a rash, weeping, or pimples, papules, or other lesions. Notify proper persons (in radiation

Nursing Interventions	**Rationales**
	department) if lesions or color changes develop.
Monitor the patient for response to analgesics and development of side effects.	Side effects of many medications include headache, nausea, vomiting, constipation, and at times, diarrhea. Side effects of codeine include headache, constipation, and nausea.
If patient is receiving chemotherapy, monitor for effects and side effects.	Effects of chemotherapeutic agents, (cyclophosphamide (Cytoxan), melphalan (Alkeran), chlorambucil (Leukeran), and carmustine (BCNU) include reduction in plasma cells and increased serum uric acid levels from cell destruction. Side effects of the chemotherapeutic agents include alopecia, nausea, vomiting, bone marrow depression leading to decreased white blood cells, decreased red blood cells, thrombocytopenia, increased chance of infection, anemia, increased possibility of bleeding, and hemorrhagic cystitis from cyclophosphamide.
Increase fluid intake to 3,000–4,000 mL daily.	Increasing intake increases excretion of excess uric acid and lessens effects on renal tissues by chemotherapy agents.
Be alert to changes in patient's behaviors related to chronic pain: withdrawal from social contacts and usual roles, sadness, crying, anger, hostility, wincing, or other behaviors.	Chronic pain not only encompasses physical pain but also has social, psychologic, and spiritual overtones. All factors must be considered in pain control efforts.
Consult proper health team members (pharmacist, anesthesiologist, clergy, and/or psychologist) to assist with pain management.	Nurses may coordinate efforts of health team in the management of the patient's pain, but various members of the health team have expertise to offer guidance for a specific patient's pain, with the goal to control the patient's pain.

DISCHARGE PLANNING/CONTINUITY OF CARE

- Coordinate with proper companies or individuals to secure needed special beds, braces or other orthoses, dietary or nutritional additives, or other special needs in time to have all supplies ready for home care.
- Complete the continuity-of-care referral in time that the home visit will be as soon after discharge as feasible.
- Provide written lists of medications, dosages, and side effects; review carefully with patient and family.
- Consult with social workers for needed supplies or assistance with ongoing financial needs.

Clinical Clip

The incidence of multiple myeloma is three times greater than all other malignant tumors of bone combined (Cipriano & McCance, 1990).

REFERENCES

Cipriano, P. F., & McCance, K. L. (1990). Alterations of leukocyte, lymphoid, and hemostatic function. In K. L. McCance & S. E. Huether (Eds.), *Pathophysiology*. St. Louis: Mosby.

Clark, J. C., & McGee, R. F. (1992). *Core curriculum for oncology nursing* (2nd ed.). Philadelphia: Saunders.

Dunbar, C. E., & Nienhuis, A. W. (1993). Multiple myeloma, new approaches to therapy. *Journal of American Medical Association, 269*(18), 2412–2416.

Lewis, S. M., & Collier, I. C. (1992). *Medical-surgical nursing* (3rd ed). St. Louis: Mosby-Yearbook.

Surgical Procedures for Orthopaedic Conditions

Surgery is a major treatment modality for orthopaedic conditions, varying from treatments for ligaments or muscle injuries to those involving bone fractures, bone tumors, degenerative conditions of joints or vertebrae, and meniscal injuries. The surgery may be performed in an outpatient setting, same-day surgical suite, or hospital operating room. The patient may be discharged within hours after the surgery or may be hospitalized for 10 days or longer, depending on the type and extent of the surgical procedure. The following care plans focus on many of the surgical procedures for orthopaedic conditions.

OPEN REDUCTION WITH INTERNAL FIXATION DEVICES

Open reductions are done because of the inability to bring about a closed reduction of the fractured bones, the need to create a more stable reduction, or the need to reduce and fix several fractured bones. Once reduced and anatomically aligned as nearly normal as possible, the fracture sites are held by internal fixation devices, including screws, pins, nails, rods, prostheses, compression plates with screws, and bone grafts.

ETIOLOGIES

- Accident causing unstable fracture of one or more bones
- Congenital anomaly causing slipping, as in spondylolisthesis
- Fall, causing fracture of one or more bones of the upper or lower extremity or of the hip
- Unstable fracture of femur or other bone

CLINICAL MANIFESTATIONS

- Acute pain in involved area after initial numbness
- Deformity of involved bone(s)
- Inability to bear weight
- Inability to use affected part(s) normally
- Internal or external rotation of affected bone
- Shortening and/or overriding of distal fracture fragments
- Soft tissue trauma, such as edema, bruising, and coolness

CLINICAL/DIAGNOSTIC FINDINGS

- Acute pain in affected area
- History of accident or fall or of congenital anomaly
- Physical examination elicits deformity, shortening, change in function, numbness, bruising, and edema

- Roentgenograms, computerized tomography (CT), or magnetic resonance imaging (MRI) shows fracture of one or more bones with rotation and overriding or slippage of vertebra from normal position

▶ NURSING DIAGNOSIS: *Acute Pain*

Related To fracture(s) of one or more bones and soft tissue injury

Defining Characteristics

- Diaphoresis
- Grimacing, moaning, crying, or rocking
- Guarding or holding affected part
- Restlessness
- Verbalizes having severe pain and discomfort
- Verbalizes inability to use part normally

Patient Outcomes

The patient will

- experience relief of pain with treatments.
- regain use of affected tissues after treatments and healing.

Nursing Interventions	Rationales
Assess pain characteristics: location, type, severity, quality, onset, duration, and alleviating or exacerbating factors.	Data are necessary for planning individualized care. Pain is usually severe with movement of part(s) and is continuous.
Maintain support and immobilization of affected part.	Closed reduction may have been previously attempted without full success, necessitating surgical correction. The affected part may be held in a splint or cast temporarily.
Elevate the affected area. Remember: *R*est, *I*ce, *C*ompression, *E*levation.	Elevation lessens edema by increasing venous return.
Apply ice bags or cold therapy to area.	Ice causes vasoconstriction to lessen bleeding as well as relieving pain.
Administer analgesia, if appropriate.	Analgesia relieves pain and lessens anxiety and restlessness. The analgesic may be given as a preoperative medication, along with a drug to lessen secretions.

Nursing Interventions	Rationales
Prepare patient for diagnostic examinations; assist as needed.	Prior to surgical reduction and internal fixation, the patient will undergo a physician's visit to secure a medical history, history of the injury, physical examination, blood work, roentgen studies and urinalysis, preoperative prescriptions, and other studies as needed.
Prepare the patient for surgery when requested.	Surgery may be performed immediately after stabilization in the emergency suite if the patient's condition warrants. It may be delayed for 1–3 days to secure definitive diagnostic studies or to allow the patient a longer stabilization period. It may also be delayed for 1–10 days or longer if the patient is not able to reach proper medical facilities or if the local tissues at the fracture site have blisters or other skin condition that could complicate surgical incisions or predispose to infection.
Inspect skin surfaces for open areas, presence of blisters, or presence of other lesions.	Fracture blisters occur at fracture sites often related to lack of reduction of the fracture or to compression that is too snug. Eczema or skin rash of various etiologies may also prevent immediate surgical reduction if in the operative site.

▶ NURSING DIAGNOSIS: *Impaired Physical Mobility*

Related To internal fixation with

- compression plate(s) with screws
- hip pinning with multiple pins or hip nail with or without side plate
- spinal fusion with bone grafts and retention screws
- insertion of intramedullary rod with transfixing pin
- insertion of endoprosthesis following removal of fractured femoral head
- insertion of spinal rods, such as Harrington, Cotrel-Dubousset, or Luque rods

Defining Characteristics

- Bedrest
- Decreased muscle strength
- Mechanical restriction of movement (pins, immobilization device, cast)
- Operative report with open reduction with internal fixation (ORIF)
- Physician's postoperative diagnosis with operative report stating insertion of one of the internal fixators listed above
- Postoperative prescriptions related to bedrest, position, and such

Patient Outcomes

The patient will

- regain ambulation with ambulatory aid as prescribed.
- regain mobility after bone healing without limp or limitation.
- regain muscle strength and coordination after treatments and healing.

Nursing Interventions	Rationales
Maintain proper position in bed as prescribed.	Commonly, patients are in dorsal recumbent position in bed.
Adjust position q2–3h; use pillows to back and between legs if appropriate; use logrolling if spinal fusion done or spinal rods have been inserted. Keep abduction pillow in place if prosthesis was inserted into femur.	Turning and position changes aid circulation, lessen muscle fatigue, and give patient a sense of well-being. Logrolling requires that the patient's spinal column does not or is not twisted until bone grafts, if used, heal. Initially two nursing personnel are needed as the patient should be passive during logrolling. As strength is regained, the patient can actively participate during logrolling so long as the back is not twisted. An abduction pillow is shaped like an A to help keep the operative limb in an abducted position to help hold the prosthesis in the acetabulum.
Elevate upper or lower extremity on pillow.	Elevation aids venous return to decrease edema formation.
Apply ice to site of surgery.	Ice decreases bleeding and lessens pain.

Nursing Interventions	Rationales
Encourage active range-of-motion (ROM) exercises to unaffected joints, such as flexion and extension exercises.	Range-of-motion exercises help maintain strength in nonaffected muscles.
Encourage use of trapeze, if permitted, to help adjust bed positions.	Using a trapeze helps the patient lift and move self.
When allowed up, assist patient to be up in chair, with partial or full weight bearing as prescribed; lift or support operative limb if needed during moving out of bed.	A patient may be allowed up the night of surgery, the first postoperative day, or after 3 or more postoperative days, depending on site of injury, associated injuries, or coexisting diseases or conditions. Weight bearing may be partial after insertion of hip nails or prostheses or intramedullary rods to thigh or non–weight bearing after tibial or fibular internal fixation. Bones of the upper extremity may be held in a sling when up. Support operative limb under joints above and below operative site; avoid pressure on soft tissues.
Assist the patient with use of a cane, walker, or crutches.	Because of weight-bearing limitations or muscle weakness, the patient may use an ambulatory aid.
Seek consultation with physical therapist for assistance with ambulation as needed.	Specialists provide assistance with specific ambulation techniques.

▶ NURSING DIAGNOSIS: *Impaired Gas Exchange*

Related To general anesthesia and bedrest

Defining Characteristics

- Has shallow, rapid respiratory patterns
- Was anesthetized for 2 or more h
- Has ineffective cough
- On prescribed bedrest

Patient Outcomes

The patient will

- cough effectively to produce clear sputum.
- regain full, deep respiratory patterns.
- regain clear breath sounds.
- not develop atelectasis or pneumonia.

Nursing Interventions	Rationales
Assess respiratory patterns, rates, depth, and breath sounds q1–3 h.	Anesthesia, especially general inhalation types, decreases respirations and irritates lungs. Breath sounds should be heard clearly in all lobes of lungs. Bedrest lowers respiratory excursions, especially when flat in bed.
Encourage deep-breathing exercises and coughing, if permitted, q2–3h.	Deep breathing lowers the diaphragm to increase inhalation of oxygen and exchange of carbon dioxide. Coughing clears secretions from respiratory tree. Sputum should be clear but may be initially blood tinged if endotracheal tube had been used during surgery.
Encourage use of incentive spirometry q2h.	Use of incentive spirometry forces air into alveoli to promote gas exchange. Goals should be increased as the patient's strength increases with the spirometer.
Check vital signs and temperature q1–4h initially; check temperature q4h for first 24 h or longer postoperative.	Vital signs give indications of the patient's recovery from the anesthesia and fluid balances. Blood pressures may be initially lower than normal but should return to normal ranges in 4–6 h. Pulse and respiratory rates may be higher than normal because of anesthetic or blood loss. They should also slow to nearer normal rates in 4–8 h. Temperature readings may be low initially related to cool postanesthesia recovery rooms. Temperature

Nursing Interventions	Rationales
	rises in the 99.6 F (37.5 C) range for first postoperative day are related to inflammatory changes. Persistent temperature readings above 100 F (37.8 C) are indicative of infection somewhere in the body, such as in the lungs, urinary tract, or wound.

► NURSING DIAGNOSIS: *Impaired Skin Integrity*

Related To incision for insertion of internal fixation devices

Defining Characteristics

- Bedrest with operative limb elevated or bedrest related to spinal fusion (incision on back)
- Incision closed with skin clips
- Internal metallic fixation devices
- Redness around incision (stage of wound healing)
- Soft tissue bruising, discoloration, and edema
- Soreness, discomfort, and pain in incisional area and around bruises

Patient Outcomes

The patient will

- have well-healed incisional area and scar without keloid formation.
- have intact internal fixation devices without loosening.
- have regression (disappearance) of soft tissue bruising with no dystrophic changes.

Nursing Interventions	Rationales
Assess incisional area for normal inflammatory wound healing changes such as redness for first 1–3 days, serosanguineous drainage, edema, pain or discomfort, and intactness of skin clips; assess soft tissue bruises for color changes, edema, tenderness, discomfort or pain in area, and open areas.	Wounds and bruises go through normal inflammatory changes for varying periods up to months. Bone healing may not be complete for years until the bone has gone through remodeling (see page 19 for bone healing stages in Table 1.3) even with internal fixation devices.

Nursing Interventions	Rationales
Check edges of cast, if present, for rough areas or tight areas causing pressure on skin and underlying tissues.	Rough areas or casts that are too tight can cause breaks in the skin as well as rubbing and pressure areas in tight areas of cast.
Elevate operative limb.	Elevation increases venous return to lessen edema and venous stasis, which could lead to skin breakdown.
Apply ice or cold therapy to bruised area.	Ice decreases bleeding through vasoconstriction and lessens edema and venous stasis, decreasing potential for skin breakdown.
Reposition patient q2–3h; use pillows strategically.	Studies have shown that ischemic changes can begin in as few as 2 h if patients cannot or are not moved or repositioned, leading to potential for decubitus formation. Pillows help maintain desired positions for patients.
Observe incisional area for increase in drainage, change in color of drainage, development of hematoma, wound abscess, or odor to drainage.	These are all signs of a wound infection and should be recorded and reported to the surgeon. Wound cultures may be obtained of the drainage.
Check patient's vital signs and temperature; note any complaints of chills or color changes in skin (skin may become very red or grayish in color).	Spiking body temperatures with chills may be indicative of bacteremia or septicemia. Gram positive sepsis is noted by marked skin flushing due to exotoxins' effects on capillary sphincters, whereas gram negative sepsis is accompanied by grayish color of skin, from the effects of endotoxins on the capillary sphincters. Pulse and respirations will increase, and blood pressure readings show drops, at times to shock (systolic pressure below 80 mm Hg) levels in septicemia.

Nursing Interventions	Rationales
Use devices such as air mattresses, bed pads, heel and elbow protectors, or at times, special beds.	Such equipment and supplies distribute pressure to lessen forces on smaller areas to decrease chances of developing pressure areas or decubiti.
Use care when moving patient up in bed or when repositioning.	Shearing forces may break fragile capillaries predisposing to decubitus formation.
Check bony prominences and contiguous areas for signs of color changes: may be reddened or white.	The first stage of decubitus formation is redness due to capillary breakdown followed by whiteness from lack of circulation.
Massage *around* bony prominences several times daily.	Massage around prominences increases circulation to lessen chance of decubitus formation. Massage *over* bony prominences or reddened areas may increase capillary fragility or breakdown and hasten development of decubitus formation.
Keep bed linens dry and unwrinkled.	Wet or damp and wrinkled linens can cause skin maceration and lead to skin breakdown. Older and elderly patients have age-related skin changes such as decreased local blood flow, thinning of the epithelial layers, compromised thermoregulation, waste clearance, and nutrient transport, which put them at risk for the development of decubiti, skin tears, tape burns, abrasions, slow wound healing, and infection (Resinck, 1992).
Provide wound care, as prescribed.	Initially, following open reduction and internal fixation, the wound is covered with a gauze/cotton pad dressing held in place with adhesive strips. After 1–3 days, the dressing is removed, with the wound left open to air, or re-covered with smaller amounts of dressings,

Nursing Interventions	Rationales
	primarily depending on the presence and amount of drainage and physician's preference. Any wound suction drain is usually removed in 2–3 days with the catheter exit site covered to contain subsequent drainage. Skin sutures or clips are cleansed with antiseptic to remove any drainage and dried with sterile applicators. The wound is examined for healing, and findings are recorded for continuity and safety in care. Occasionally patients request a small dressing to cover the wound to prevent contact with their clothing and to make the wound less visible. Also, occlusive dressings may be used for some wounds to aid healing, with these dressings being transparent and occlusive and made of polymers or polyurethane that is moisture vapor permeable and able to absorb wound drainage.
Assist or remove skin sutures or clips, as prescribed, according to hospital policy.	Skin sutures or skin clips are usually removed 5–7 days or later, depending on appearance and evidence of wound healing. All wound edges should be approximated with no open or draining areas. Every other skin clip may be removed in 1 day followed by the remainder being removed the following day. Skin sutures are usually all removed on the same day. Retention or stay sutures may not be removed for up to 3 weeks or longer after surgery to help assure good collagen formation and fairly secure wound healing. Registered nurses may remove sutures and clips if these activities are within hospital policies.

Nursing Interventions	Rationales
Explain to patient to wash wound area with soap and water and to dry wound well.	Cleansing, rinsing, and drying help remove secretions or drainage and remove bacteria, lessening chance of wound infection and increasing circulation to aid wound healing.
Explain wound healing and scar formation to patient.	Learning steps eases patient's concerns. Stages or steps are (1) inflammatory, for 1–5 days with signs of gradually decreasing redness, soreness or tenderness, edema, drainage, and temperature elevation (locally at wound), all due to phagocytosis and inflammation; (2) collagen deposition, beginning on the second to third days, reaching a peak around postoperative days 12–14, (collagen is deposited and replaced daily, giving the wound strength and resistance to dehiscence); (3) wound maturation and scar formation, from initial period to 1–2 months or longer; and (4) scar contraction, during which scar shrinks in size and becomes white. Scars are avascular, with less tensile (stretch) nature when contraction is complete, which may take 3 or more months.

▶ NURSING DIAGNOSIS: *Altered Nutrition—Less Than Body Requirements*

Related To diagnostic regimen, anesthesia, and decreased postoperative intake

Defining Characteristics

- Anorexia, nausea, or vomiting
- Being held nothing by mouth (NPO) for hours and, at times, for more than 1 day
- Dislike for "clear" liquids or other foods offered
- Lack of exercise or energy expenditure
- Lower serum levels of total protein, albumin, and globulin levels

- Prolonged intravenous therapy
- Prolonged wound/bone healing

Patient Outcomes

The patient will

- begin to regain lost body weight before discharge to home.
- have sufficient intake of proteins, carbohydrates, and vitamins to stop losing weight.
- have intake of oral fluids to 3,000 mL/day.
- lose only 5–10 lb during illness and convalescent periods.
- regain appetite within 3–5 days postoperatively.
- regain muscle mass and strength.
- regain serum protein levels within normal limits (WNL).
- retain ingested foods without nausea or vomiting.

Nursing Interventions	Rationales
Assess daily intake of prescribed diet during diagnostic period; note length of time being NPO and presence of intravenous therapy.	Some diagnostic examinations do not require withholding foods or fluids. Others, such as a myelogram, require withholding them after a clear liquid breakfast. Intravenous therapy with 5% dextrose solution only replaces 200 cal/L; thus intake is below suggested dietary levels for adults.
Discuss food likes and dislikes; consult dietitian for substitutes within daily menus.	Patients generally will eat more of foods they like. Substitutions can usually be made within daily menus to meet a patient's needs or likes.
Seek physician's prescription for antinauseant medication and administer as needed or prescribed.	Some medications, especially narcotics, produce nausea and, at times, vomiting, as do some anesthetics. Antinauseant medications lessen these reactions. Narcotic medications may need to be changed to decrease episodes of nausea and vomiting.
Explain lack of appetite and discuss regaining it over time.	Appetite decreases with bedrest and injury and as part of the stress response. After the initial alarm reaction, when appetite decreases, it begins to increase during the resistance (second-phase) reaction

Nursing Interventions	Rationales
	and should be fully regained by the third (exhaustion) phase of the stress response. Also, lack of energy expenditure lowers appetite.
Discuss daily need for proteins, carbohydrates, limited fats, and high vitamin intake from foods.	Proteins with all necessary amino acids, referred to as complete proteins, help in cellular and tissue synthesis. Carbohydrates serve as fuel for protein metabolism. Fats aid satiety value and thus decrease appetite. Vitamins, especially A, C, and D, aid bone and cellular healing and vitamin B complexes aid nerve functions. Sufficient calcium should also be taken to promote strong bone formation.
Encourage intake of 3,000 mL of fluids daily.	Fluids maintain fluid balances in body, aid digestion and elimination, and help maintain circulation.
Monitor laboratory data for effects of intake on serum levels of proteins, electrolytes, and enzymes.	Levels should return to WNL as food intake is properly metabolized and utilized within body cells. Weight gain will be slow but should increase as activity, mobility, and energy expenditure increase until lost weight is regained.

▶ NURSING DIAGNOSIS: *High Risk for Infection*

Risk Factors

- Decreased immune response related to concomitant diseases
- Insertion of internal fixation devices
- Open fracture, present with some fractures
- Open wound at time of surgery

Patient Outcomes

The patient will

- experience no infection postoperatively.
- regain a well-functioning immune system.

Nursing Interventions	Rationales
Assess for presence of concomitant diseases.	Common orthopaedic diseases that decrease functions of the immune system include rheumatoid arthritis, systemic lupus erythematosus, ankylosing spondylitis, and progressive systemic sclerosis. Other diseases, such as diabetes, blood dyscrasias, and renal diseases, also lessen functions of the immune system.
Monitor vital signs and temperatures q4h for first 2–4 days postoperatively.	Changes in vital signs indicating infection include increased pulse and respiratory rates, spiking temperatures, chills, changes in sensorium or consciousness, and elevated white blood cell levels.
Monitor wound site q4–6h.	Signs of a wound infection include marked redness, increased tenderness or pain, presence of a wound abscess, or increased drainage. Another type of infection seen in orthopaedic patients with open fractures is gas gangrene, in which anaerobic organisms produce gas bubbles in the infected tissues, which produce pressure and gangrenous changes in cells, along with a putrid odor of dead cells.
Perform wound care as prescribed using wound precautions if drainage is present. Use aseptic technique for wound care.	Precautions must be taken not to make the patient's infectious process worse as well as to prevent spread of infection to other patients. Meticulous hand washing is also necessary, as is use of sterile technique and articles.
Administer tetanus antitoxin or tetanus toxoid as prescribed.	Tetanus antitoxin provides antibodies for passive immunization, and tetanus toxoid provides toxoid for building active immunity. Tetanus organisms are found in soils and dirt that could contaminate an open fracture site.

Nursing Interventions	Rationales
Administer antibiotics as prescribed.	Antibiotics may be given prophylactically if there is a high probability of an infection developing and are given therapeutically if an infection develops. Antibiotics must be given properly to maintain therapeutic blood levels.
Prepare patient for wound/joint sialogram or other diagnostic study as prescribed.	A sialogram is injection of dye along a fistulous track to determine extent of infection. At times, the metallic devices may have to be removed to help eradicate the infection.

▶ NURSING DIAGNOSIS: *High Risk for Injury (Development of Thrombophlebitis)*

Risk Factors
- Bedrest for extended periods
- Elderly or older patient
- Presence of varicose veins or injury to veins
- Venous stasis secondary to edema

Patient Outcomes
The patient will
- be relieved of edema.
- not develop thrombophlebitis.
- regain ambulatory status in early postoperative period.
- regain venous integrity.

Nursing Interventions	Rationales
Assess extremities for presence of edema, varicose veins, soreness, or tenderness along peripheral veins; perform Homan sign by dorsiflexing foot on calf.	Tenderness, edema, redness, and hot area along vein(s) are signs of thrombophlebitis, as is a positive Homan sign. This sign is positive if there is increased pain with dorsiflexion of foot along superficial veins or deep in calf muscle. Rarely

Nursing Interventions	Rationales
	does the area develop cyanosis or lose sensation. Pain may be mild to moderate with acute thrombophlebitis.
Maintain bedrest with affected extremity elevated.	Bedrest lessens metabolic demands on tissues, and elevation decreases edema and increases venous return.
Apply antiembolism hose, if prescribed.	These elasticized hose constrict superficial veins so blood is channeled to deeper veins, lessening superficial venous stasis.
Apply intermittent pulsating pressure equipment to legs as prescribed.	This form of treatment creates muscle compressions through alternating pressures to increase circulation and lessen venous stasis.
Administer low-dose or low-molecular-weight heparin as prescribed.	Heparin prevents formation of clots by interrupting the clotting process.
Encourage ankle flexion/extension exercises.	Flexion/extension exercises increase muscle contractions to lessen venous stasis.
Administer aspirin as prescribed.	Aspirin interferes with the clotting process, thereby decreasing clot formation.
Prepare patient for blood flow studies, if done.	Studies of venous blood flow such as plethysmography, venogram, and ultrasound help determine presence or absence of clots in the peripheral veins studied.
Monitor laboratory studies related to blood clotting, such as prothrombin time or partial thromboplastin studies.	Serial studies of these two tests provide data relative to adequacy of therapeutic measures as well as alerting health team to needed changes to prevent gross bleeding or clot formation.

▶ NURSING DIAGNOSIS: *Knowledge Deficit*

Related To sudden injury, unfamiliar terms, and shock

Defining Characteristics

- Lack of familiarity with terms
- Misconceptions from past experiences
- Unfamiliarity with multiple "strange-named" diagnostic tests
- Necessity of surgical repair
- Severity of trauma leading to shock
- Sudden, unexpected injury

Patient Outcomes

The patient will

- be able to participate actively in decision-making process.
- develop understanding of severity, extent, and proposed treatments of trauma.

Nursing Interventions	Rationales
Assess understanding of condition, diagnostic examinations, and proposed treatments after physician's explanations.	Because of shock, unfamiliar terms, or other reasons, the patient may have incomplete understanding of the treatment plan.
Ask questions to determine what additional information patient wants.	Answers to the questions determine the teaching plan.
Use charts, diagrams, or pictures to clarify patient's understandings.	Multiple techniques aid the learning process, as persons learn in different patterns.
Stress patient's activities (turning, exercises, and such) to prevent complications.	Because of lack of previous injuries of similar nature, the patient needs specific instructions for active participation.
Teach patient how to use an ambulatory aid, if needed.	Specific instructions are needed for use of each type of aid.
Teach patient how to apply elastic hose, if to be used.	Proper application of elastic hose is required for safe use.
Teach patient expected and side effects of medications.	Learning what is expected lessens anxiety. Learning the side effects

Nursing Interventions	Rationales
	helps patient accept them when they occur or consult with physician for a change in medication.
Teach patient self-care, as needed.	Knowing how to do own care lessens anxiety.
Provide written instructions prior to discharge.	Having written instructions provides a safety factor that the patient will not forget vital information.

DISCHARGE PLANNING/CONTINUITY OF CARE

- Refer to home care nurses for wound care, nutritional assistance and assistance with activities of daily living as needed.
- Refer to physical therapist for assistance with ambulation and exercise regimen.
- Provide written guidelines for medications, their purposes, and side effects.
- Secure follow-up physician's appointment.

Clinical Clip

More than 280,000 hip fractures occurred in the United States in 1993, more than 760 a day (Robb, 1993).

Clinical Clip

After age 50, fracture rates in women are two to three times greater than in men. Among men, hip fracture rates increase significantly only after age 85 (Robb, 1993).

Clinical Clip

The number of persons aged 65 and older is increasing two and a half times faster than the overall population. The number of persons aged 85 and older is increasing six times faster than the overall population (Robb, 1993).

Clinical Clip

Risk Factors

Gender

Heredity: white and Asian women are one and a half to two times more likely to have hip fractures than African-American or Hispanic women

Chronic medical diseases

Visual impairment

Muscle weakness

Balance and gait disorder

Improper nutrition

Extrinsic: medications, smoking, excessive alcohol consumption, home and environmental hazards, institutional hazards

REFERENCES

Kim, M. J., McFarland, G. K., & McLane, A. M. (1993). *Pocket guide to nursing diagnoses* (5th ed.). St. Louis: Mosby-Yearbook.

Mourad, L. A. (1991). *Orthopedic disorders.* St. Louis, MO: Mosby-Yearbook.

Mourad, L. A., & Droste, M. (1993). *The nursing care of adults with orthopaedic conditions* (3rd ed.). Albany: Delmar.

Nogalski, M. P., & Bach, B. R. Jr. (1993). A review of early anterior cruciate ligament surgical repair or reconstruction. *Orthopaedic Review, 22*(11), 1213–1222.

Resnick, B. (1992). Wound care in the elderly. *Reflections, 18*(4), 18.

Robb, W. J. III. (1993). Hip fracture disease: Coping with a contemporary epidemic. *Journal of Musculoskeletal Medicine, 10*(12), 12–24.

Salmond, S. W., Mooney, N. E., & Verdisco, L. A. (1991). *Core curriculum for orthopaedic nursing* (2nd ed.). Pitman, NJ: Jannetti.

Shaw, J. A., & Wilson, S. (1993). Internal fixation of proximal femur fractures: A biomechanical comparison of the gamma locking nail and the omega compression hip screw. *Orthopaedic Review, 22*(1), 61–68.

Total Joint Replacements

Total joint replacements involve replacing both surfaces of the bones in a joint. Theoretically, all joints can be replaced when technology is able to develop and perfect the prosthetic parts. Currently, however, joints of the hip, knee, shoulder, ankle, elbow, wrist, and fingers are the joints which are replaced. Approximately 150,000–280,000 hip joints and 125,000–150,000 knee joints are replaced yearly, many of which are due to the degenerative changes of osteoarthritis, rheumatoid arthritis, or fractures of the hip. Shoulder joints are also replaced fairly frequently.

Elbow, wrist, and ankle replacements are done much less frequently and with less success. Occasionally after several replacements of wrists or ankles, these joints may require an arthrodesis (joint fusion) because of lack of remaining bone surfaces or bone stock. Research is ongoing regarding all joint replacement prostheses, but the operation affords increased mobility, freedom from pain, and a much more positive outlook for the majority of persons having hip, knee, or shoulder replacements.

TOTAL HIP REPLACEMENT

Uncemented arthroplasties involve the use of bioingrowth prostheses, which promote bone growth on their surfaces through the use of beaded surfaces, grooves, metallic/polyethylene surfaces, screws, and "press fit" to help hold the prostheses more firmly in the joints. Many total hip replacements begin loosening in approximately 10 years and require replacement arthroplasty, with both parts needing replacement or just one side. Newer technology also has developed prosthetic parts with a femoral component without an attached "head," so that if the femoral stem is intact and solidly seated in the femoral shaft, only the head or the acetabular portions may need to be replaced. Conversely, possibly only the femoral shaft prosthesis requires replacement, with the other prostheses remaining intact.

ETIOLOGIES

- Avascular necrosis of femoral head and acetabulum
- Fracture of femur and/or acetabulum leading to degenerative changes
- Osteoarthritis of hip joint

CLINICAL MANIFESTATIONS

- Decreased range-of-motion (ROM) of hip joint
- Inability to use hip joint normally and to bear full weight
- Limp
- Persistent pain in hip joint, especially at night

CLINICAL/DIAGNOSTIC FINDINGS

- History of increasing pain in hip joint(s) over time and past history of fractured acetabulum or ankylosing spondylitis or osteoarthritis
- Physical examination revealing marked limitation of joint movement, tight hip muscles, and tenderness in hip joint on palpation; no redness present
- Roentgenograms showing decreased joint space, loss of joint cartilage, presence of bone cysts and osteophytes (bone spurs), or avascular necrosis

- Roentgenograms showing old fracture of acetabulum or fracture of femoral head or neck
- Serologic studies showing negative rheumatoid factor, positive human leukocyte antigen (HLA) B27, hemoglobin of 13 g, and hematocrit of 39%

▶ NURSING DIAGNOSIS: *Impaired Physical Mobility*

Related To degenerative changes in hip joint

Defining Characteristics

- Presence of limp when weight bearing
- ROM of joint limited
- Roentgenogram findings as given above

Patient Outcomes

The patient will

- regain mobility without limp or leg length discrepancy.
- regain satisfactory ROM after total joint replacement.
- retain muscle functions within normal limits.
- retain prostheses within hip joint/capsule with use.

Nursing Interventions	Rationales
Assess for position of operative limb.	Operative limb is kept in abducted position with an abduction pillow to help hold the prostheses within the joint.
Reposition patient q2h.	The patient may be on bedrest on operative day but may be prescribed to be turned to unoperative side to help maintain circulation. Some physicians want the patient to lie on the back only, and some allow the patient to be turned to the operative side.
Assist patient to do ROM exercises to unaffected joints.	Range-of-motion exercises help muscles and joints maintain normal strength and functions.
Complete referral for physical therapy.	Physical therapy techniques help the patient regain functions of operative joint and muscles as well

Nursing Interventions	Rationales
	as assist patient to retain normal functions in unaffected joints.
Assist physical therapist to get patient up to a chair, when allowed up.	Usually the patient is allowed up on postoperative day 1 or 2, with transfer to a chair for sitting upright. The legs are to remain uncrossed and the feet kept on the floor.
Assist the physical therapist to ambulate the patient.	The patient may begin ambulation on postoperative day 4 or 5 using a walker to aid ambulation. The patient may bear weight on the operative hip to the point of pain. He or she may be gotten up several or more times a day to ambulate. When sitting, the hip is not to be flexed beyond 90° to prevent dislodging the prostheses.
Teach patient to use walker and crutches.	The patient will initially use a walker, adjusted to the proper height, but will probably go home using crutches until roentgenograms show sufficient healing (6 weeks to 3 months for crutches). The walker or crutches provide stability and safety for the patient.
Teach patient plantar flexion and dorsiflexion exercises of both ankles, plus other tightening exercises as prescribed, e.g., quadriceps setting exercises.	Ankle exercises help maintain circulation to prevent development of thrombi and thrombophlebitis. Quadriceps setting helps maintain strength in thigh muscles needed for walking and weight bearing.
Teach patient to wear well-fitting footwear.	Properly fitting footwear provides stability and security when ambulating.
Teach patient to increase ambulation as per physician's prescription.	Ambulation is gradually increased over time as strength and healing progress (x-rays show bioingrowth and stability as needed).

▶ NURSING DIAGNOSIS: *Impaired Gas Exchange*

Related To bedrest, anesthesia, or chronic lung condition, such as emphysema

Defining Characteristics

- Bedrest prescribed for 2 postoperative days
- Preoperative chest x-ray shows no lung infection but presence of mild emphysema
- Underwent general inhalation anesthesia for arthroplasty

Patient Outcomes

The patient will

- have no pulmonary infection.
- reach goals for incentive spirometry.
- regain normal levels of respiratory functions.

Nursing Interventions	Rationales
Assess respiratory rates, breath sounds, and cough.	An increased respiratory rate may be one indication of a developing respiratory infection. Decreased breath sounds and a cough signify presence of secretions in pulmonary tissues.
Monitor vital signs and body temperature.	A pulmonary infection may be noted by elevated temperatures, pulse, and respiratory rates, especially in first 24–48 h postoperative after inhalation anesthesia.
Listen to breath sounds in all lobes of both lungs q4h.	Breath sounds should be heard clearly in all lobes of both lungs. Inability to hear breath sounds may signify atelectasis or presence of secretions blocking passage of air.
Encourage deep breathing and cough q4h.	Deep breathing helps perfusion of alveoli and aids in exchange of oxygen and carbon dioxide. If cough is productive of yellow or green sputum, a lung or bronchial infection may be present.
Encourage use of incentive spirometer q2–3h; encourage patient to reach established goals.	Incentive spirometry increases lung expansion to lessen chance of infection.

Nursing Interventions	Rationales
Assist patient to turn in bed and to be up, when allowed.	Turning from back to side facilitates circulation and perfusion through lung tissues. Ambulation increases deep breathing and lung perfusion.
If emphysema is marked or pronounced, teach patient pursed lip and abdominal breathing exercises.	Pursed lip breathing involves exhaling against resistance, which helps keep alveoli open to aid oxygen exchange. Abdominal breathing forces diaphragm lower to bring more oxygen into lungs.

▶ NURSING DIAGNOSIS: *Acute Pain*

Related To surgical trauma and incision

Defining Characteristics

- Complains of much soreness in back, operative leg, and muscles
- Has a 6–8-in. incision on upper lateral thigh closed with skin clips and covered with a dressing
- Has pain in operative area, partially relieved by use of patient-controlled analgesia (PCA) pump with morphine or other narcotic as the analgesic
- Presence of epidural catheter for pain control

Patient Outcomes

The patient will

- have a well-healed incision without infection or wound separation.
- regain a relatively pain-free state after wound healing.

Nursing Interventions	Rationales
Assess presence, sites, duration, intensity, and type of pain.	Individuals have different pain thresholds and pain experiences. Assessment data should indicate adequacy of pain relief or need for change.
Monitor use and effects of PCA solution q4h.	Determines how often and what effects the medication is having. It may be necessary to adjust the

Nursing Interventions	Rationales
	type of medication and the dosage for a specific patient.
Assist patient to adjust positions q2h.	Adjusting positions frequently eases tired, sore muscles and joints to aid comfort by relieving pressure on nerve endings.
Monitor injection of analgesic medication per epidural catheter, if being used. (Management of injections via the epidural catheter is usually by the acute-pain service of the hospital.)	Some patients may have epidural catheters for pain relief rather than using a PCA pump or injectable narcotics.
Perform neurovascular checks q2h.	Increased pain noted during neurovascular checks may signify increasing venous pressure, bleeding into tissues, thrombophlebitis, or other complication requiring additional checks or care.
Perform wound care as prescribed, noting any drainage, redness, increased tenderness, or pain in incisional area.	Drainage (unless serous or serosanguineous), redness, increased tenderness, and pain are signs of a wound infection.
Teach patient pain-relieving techniques, such as visualization, relaxation techniques, diversionary activities, and others.	Since many types of pain are related to anoxia, oxygen intake and cellular distribution is enhanced by using relaxation, deep breathing, visualization, and other techniques.

▶ NURSING DIAGNOSIS: *Altered Peripheral Tissue Perfusion*

Related To surgical trauma and venous stasis

Defining Characteristics

- Has much pain and soreness in operative thigh, leg, and ankle
- Presence of marked edema in operative thigh, leg, and ankle

Patient Outcomes

The patient will

- be relieved of pain and soreness in muscles and joints.

- not develop thrombophlebitis.
- regain tissue perfusion with only a small amount of edema.

Nursing Interventions	Rationales
Assess neurovascular status in all nine parameters.	Provides data of status of perfusion of operative limb.
Apply elastic hose to both extremities (if operative limb not wrapped with elastic bandages).	Elastic hose decreases edema and constricts peripheral veins to decrease venous stasis.
Apply antithrombotic motorized intermittent pulsating system wraps to operative limb or both limbs as prescribed.	Intermittent pulsating wraps alternately apply external pressure to venous tissues to prevent stasis and lessen possibility of thrombophlebitis or thrombus formation secondary to increased venous pressure during insertion of the femoral prosthesis.
Administer low-dose heparin, low-molecular-weight heparin, or low-dose aspirin as prescribed.	Heparin and aspirin helps prevent thrombus formation.
Perform Homan sign by dorsiflexing the foot toward calf or leg.	Positive if there is pain deep in the calf muscle when the foot is dorsiflexed. Pain deep in the calf is a sign of thrombophlebitis.
Encourage active ankle flexion and extension exercises.	These exercises aid resolution of edema and increase peripheral circulation to lessen possibility of thrombophlebitis.
Assist patient to be up and ambulate as prescribed.	Ambulation aids venous return and lessens stasis.

▶ NURSING DIAGNOSIS: *High Risk for Injury*

Risk Factors

- Poor muscle/joint strength
- Uncemented prostheses on both sides of hip joint

Patient Outcomes

The patient will

- not experience dislocation of the prostheses.
- regain satisfactory muscle/joint strength.

Nursing Interventions	Rationales
Assess position of operative leg and thigh in abduction pillow.	The limb is to be maintained abducted to aid retention of the prostheses in the hip joint. The abduction pillow helps in maintaining the required position until the muscles/joint recovers from the surgical trauma.
Assist the patient to use the "post position" to lift body.	The post position involves bending the knee, firmly planting the unoperative foot on the mattress, and pushing down on the foot while lifting the body (holding it rigid) by grasping the trapeze with both hands. By lifting in this manner, the operative hip and limb are kept rigid and unflexed, which should prevent dislocation.
Assist nursing personnel to turn patient to unoperative side as prescribed, adjusting abduction pillow to support leg properly.	Turning eases tired muscles, lessens pain and soreness, and gives the patient a sense that recovery is proceeding normally. Avoid holding operative hip over surgery area during turning as pressure could possibly dislodge prostheses.
Teach patient not to cross knees or ankles.	Crossing knees or ankles involves adducting limb, which could dislodge prosthesis.
Teach patient buttocks setting exercises, along with quadriceps setting exercises.	These types of exercises strengthen the muscles which surround the hip joint to firm up and strengthen the joint.
Seek consultation with occupational therapists for assistive devices to aid	Occupational therapists assist the patient to do self-care and dressing

Nursing Interventions	Rationales
in reaching, applying socks or slippers, and such.	while using long-handled reachers and grabbers. Use of these devices prevents the patient from hyperflexing operative hip beyond 90°, which could dislodge prostheses.
Observe patient while ambulating to note amount of weight bearing (patient is usually allowed weight "to point of pain").	Because of operative trauma, the patient usually has limited weight bearing related to pain in operative site for up to 3 or more weeks, after which the patient switches from a walker to crutches when ambulating.
Teach the patient the purposes of limiting weight bearing according to physician's prescription.	Until x-rays show some bioingrowth (at 3 months or later postoperatively), the physician will limit full weight bearing.
Reiterate crutch walking techniques, sitting for no longer than 30 min, lying flat or with only 30°–45° elevation of head of bed, and if riding in the car, stopping and walking every hour.	These instructions help maintain muscle strength and safe postoperative activities to maintain the prostheses within the hip joint.

▶ NURSING DIAGNOSIS: *Impaired Skin Integrity*

Related To drain in wound, incision, and presence of skin clips or sutures

Defining Characteristics

- Incision along upper lateral surface of thigh
- Presence of suction-type wound drain
- Skin clips/sutures closing wound

Patient Outcomes

The patient will

- regain wound healing by first intention.
- have no excessive wound drainage.

Nursing Interventions	Rationales
Assess wound site, amount of drainage on dressing, and amount in suction drainage collecting receptacle.	On initial dressing change (postoperative day 2 or 3), the wound may appear slightly reddened and edematous, with coagulum around the skin clips or sutures. The dressing will contain serosanguineous drainage and the suction drainage receptacle may contain 10 or more mL. The receptacle may be prescribed to be emptied q2–4h and amount measured and recorded. The usual amount of drainage is between 100 and 200 mL total. The suction drain is usually removed on postoperative day 2 or 3 if the drainage has decreased and become static (separated serum and red blood cells noted in tubing). A small sterile dressing is used to cover the incisional area after the initial dressing is removed.
Change dressing daily and cleanse any drainage from incisional area and from skin clips or sutures using aseptic technique.	Cleansing drainage from wound prevents maceration of skin areas and lessens chance of wound infection. Aseptic technique prevents bringing pathogens to area.
Observe incisional site, skin clips/sutures for reddened areas, edema, increased drainage, or development of hematoma or abscess.	A hematoma may form due to walled-off sanguineous drainage or bleeding. An abscess is a collection of purulent material signifying a wound infection. As inflammatory changes lessen with wound healing, redness, edema, and soreness markedly decrease in 4 to 5 days postoperatively.
Remove skin clips/sutures as prescribed (if a nursing function or institution policy).	Skin clips or sutures may be removed on day 6, 7, or later depending on amount of wound healing. Every other skin clip or suture may be initially removed, followed on the next day by

Nursing Interventions	Rationales
	removal of the remaining clips or sutures. The wound is cleansed and left open to air after clip/suture removal.
Observe all skin areas and bony prominences q4–6h.	Signs of pressure areas include color changes (skin may be reddened or whiter than surrounding tissues), and the patient may complain of burning, tenderness, or numbness in a discolored area if a pressure area is developing. Skin color should not be bluish as this is a sign of venous stasis (deoxygenation) and pressure.
Massage around bony prominences q4h. Caution: Do not massage over reddened or white areas; only massage around them gently, using care not to lacerate skin with nails.	Massage increases circulation to the area and hastens removal of wastes. Reddened areas signify injury to capillaries and beginning inflammatory changes.

▶ NURSING DIAGNOSIS: *Altered Urinary Output*

Related To anesthesia, bedrest, and surgical trauma

Defining Characteristics

- Asks to be put on bed pan or use urinal
- Unable to void when bed pan/urinal in place

Patient Outcomes

The patient will

- be able to empty bladder with voiding.
- begin urinating on own on postoperative day 1.
- possibly require catheterization within 10–12 h postoperatively.

Nursing Interventions	Rationales
Assess bladder area for distention; ask patient if bladder feels full or if has urge to void.	A full bladder will be able to be palpated above the pubic symphysis. Pressure over a full bladder

Nursing Interventions	Rationales
	will usually increase the patient's need to void.
Monitor the amount of blood loss at surgery, amount replaced, and intravenous fluid replacement in previous 8–12 h.	Determining amount of fluid intake helps determine amount of fluid perfusing kidney and amount of urine formed in previous 8–12 h.
Carefully place patient on small fracture bed pan to facilitate voiding if urge to void is present 8–10 h postoperatively (or place urinal).	The urge to void develops from pressure over the trigone area in the bladder from presence of urine in bladder. Use of a small fracture bed pan (or female urinal) lessens chance of dislocating prostheses. Males usually can void in 8–10 h if fluids lost have been replaced and the prostate is not obstructing the posterior urethra. Allow patient privacy to void. Run water in the sink and have patient dangle fingers in warm water to aid voiding or pour a measured amount of water over vulva to aid opening of external sphincter to aid voiding.
Secure order to catheterize patient if unable to void after 12 h, and patient is very distended and markedly uncomfortable. Use a straight catheter and aseptic technique.	Catheterization may be needed in first 10–12 h postoperatively due to constriction of sphincters from narcotic administration, surgical trauma, and effects of anesthesia. Usually a straight catheter is used for single use only, and an indwelling catheter is not used if it is not in place after surgery. Indwelling catheters may cause a urinary tract infection.
Keep intravenous fluids infusing as prescribed while maintaining patient's nothing-by-mouth (NPO) status.	Patient's only fluid intake is from intravenous replacements, and intake should be 3,000 mL q24h to maintain fluid balances.
Encourage use of bed pan or urinal and voiding techniques to help patient void on own.	After inability to void initially, the patient may be able to void on own during awake hours and after anesthetic effects are gone.

Nursing Interventions	Rationales
Encourage patient to ask for bed pan before urgency is marked.	If patient tries to void q6–8h before bladder is too distended, he or she may be successful since urgency is not present.
When allowed oral fluids, encourage intake of 1,000 mL (if not contraindicated) q8h.	Fluid intake should be 3,000 mL q24h for proper perfusion of cells, fluid balances, and renal/urinary output.
Monitor intake and output q8h and record 24-h totals.	Recording and analyzing 8-h and 24-h totals provides data to determine if changes are needed.

NOTE: For complications after total hip replacements, see page 289.

DISCHARGE PLANNING/CONTINUITY OF CARE

- Refer to home care nurses for continuing wound care, if needed.
- Consult with social service for assistance in securing walker, toilet riser, or other supplies as needed.
- Provide written lists of medications, their purposes, and expected side effects needed for ongoing treatment of chronic conditions and for analgesia.
- Secure follow-up physician's appointment.

REFERENCES

Bargar, W. L. (1990). Preoperative planning in revision total hip replacement surgery. *Orthopaedic Review (Oct. Suppl.)*, 16–22.

Childs, S. (1993). Avascular necrosis of the bone: The causes and cure. *Orthopaedic Nursing, 12*(4), 29–34.

Head, W. C., Mallory, T. H., & Emerson, R. H. (1990). Principles of cementless acetabular reconstruction in primary and revision cases. *Orthopaedic Review (Oct. Suppl.)*, 32–37.

Maklebust, J. A. (1993). AHCPR guideline: Pressure ulcers. *Ohio Nurses Review, 68*(5), 20.

Mallory, T. J. (1993). Cement remains the best choice to fix a total hip stem. *Orthopedics Today, 12*(1), 1, 12.

Mourad, L. A., & Droste, M. (1993). *The nursing care of adults with orthopaedic conditions* (3rd ed.). Albany: Delmar.

Resinck, B. (1992). Wound care in the elderly. *Reflections, 18*(4), 8.

TOTAL KNEE REPLACEMENT

Knees are the second most frequently replaced joints after hip replacements. Total knee replacement (TKR) involves replacing the articular cartilage of the condyles of the distal femur and of the proximal tibia and fibula. As with the hip joint, metal and polyethylene prostheses are used, with the metallic prosthesis replacing the distal femoral cartilage. The majority of the knee replacements are done for osteoarthritic conditions, with some done for traumatic conditions and some for treating idiopathic conditions. Between 125,000 and 150,000 new or revision knee arthroplasties are done yearly. Also, as with the hip, one or more of the prostheses may be replaced if some of the prostheses remain intact.

Total knee replacements are done with a tourniquet applied on the distal thigh to create a bloodless environment for the surgical procedure. The incision is made anteriorly to expose the knee structures clearly. Bioingrowth prostheses are currently used with the tibial/fibular prostheses also anchored with screws for more secure attachment. Also, methyl methacrylate may be used, especially for revision of previous total knee replacements. Bone grafts may be added to the tibial and/or fibular surfaces to help assure that adequate bone stock is present. Again, as with the hip, a suction-type drainage system is used and the entire foot, leg, and thigh are dressed in a wrapping of alternating layers of elastic wrap and sheet wadding to permit some edema formation while maintaining a firm dressing. A knee immobilizer may be applied also or the operative limb may be placed in a continuous passive motion (CPM) machine for initiating passive movements when prescribed. The operative limb is elevated and cold therapy is applied to lessen edema formation and pain.

▶ NURSING DIAGNOSIS: *Impaired Physical Mobility*

Related To total knee replacement and bedrest

Defining Characteristics

- Bedrest for operative day
- Operative knee in knee immobilizer (or CPM machine)

- Replacement of articular surfaces of distal femur, proximal tibia, and fibula

Patient Outcomes

The patient will

- perform active exercises to aid rehabilitation.
- regain physical mobility with use of walker or crutches as prescribed.
- use CPM machine to exercise operative knee.

Nursing Interventions	Rationales
Assess operative limb for presence of CPM machine, long leg/thigh wrapping, or knee immobilizer, and suction drainage.	Variations in use of wrap/dressing, CPM machine, or knee immobilizer are related to whether or not knee replacement is primary or revision surgery, types of prostheses used, bone grafts in place, and physician's preference.
Perform all nine neurovascular checks q1–2h as prescribed.	It is vital that neurovascular checks be carefully done because of use of tourniquet with possibility of circulatory impairment or development of compartment syndrome (see pages 299–304).
Keep operative limb elevated as prescribed.	Elevation lessens edema formation and increases venous return.
Apply cold therapy to operative limb.	Cold constricts vessels, thereby lessening edema formation.
Observe dressing for drainage, looking under knee area; measure and empty drainage in suction chamber.	Drainage tubing may become obstructed, causing drainage to appear on dressing. Gravity will cause drainage to run or flow to behind knee area.
When allowed up (usually first postoperative day), assist patient to be in a chair with operative limb elevated.	Getting the patient up is positive as it helps the patient develop a positive outlook for optimal recovery. Elevation lessens edema formation.
Seek consultation with physical therapists for rehabilitation exercises and aid in ambulating patient.	Specialists have current knowledge and skills to aid the patient toward maximal rehabilitation and ambulation.

Nursing Interventions	Rationales
Encourage the patient to perform active exercises as prescribed.	Nurses assist patients at times that physical therapists are busy or unavailable. They must understand the types and purposes of the exercises and techniques involved.
Assist the patient to ambulate with walker, crutches, or cane(s) when allowed.	Until operative trauma is resolved and bioingrowth has begun, the patient uses an ambulatory aid for safety and security.

NOTE: The remainder of nursing interventions following total knee replacement for the same nursing diagnoses are similar to those for total hip replacement and will not be repeated to avoid redundancy. For complications after knee replacements, see page 289.

DISCHARGE PLANNING/CONTINUITY OF CARE

- Refer to physical therapy for rehabilitation exercises, crutches, and instructions for use.
- Secure appointment for follow-up physician's visit.
- Refer to home care nurses for wound care as needed.

REFERENCES

Buechel, F. F. (1990). Cemented and cementless revision arthroplasty using rotating-platform total knee implants: A 12-year experience. *Orthopaedic Review (Oct. Suppl.)*, 71–75.

Gross, A. E. (1993). Allografts effectively fill knee defects. *Orthopedic Special Edition, 2*(9), 12.

Rand, J. A., & Lai, C. H. (1993). Revision succeeds in failed UNI knees. *Orthopedic Special Edition, 2*(9), 18.

Stiehl, J. B. (1993). Implant modularity enhances revision TKA. *Orthopedic Special Edition, 2*(9), 10.

Whiteside, L. A. (1993). Morcellized bone promising in cementless TKA. *Orthopedic Special Edition, 2*(9), 11.

TOTAL SHOULDER REPLACEMENT

Shoulder replacement arthroplasty is similar to that for a hip as both joints are ball-and-socket joints. But the total shoulder has not been done as long or as often as has the hip. Total shoulder replacement (TSR) is being done more often recently as prostheses have been developed. Estimates of the frequency of TSR indicate there were 4,000 TSRs and 2,000 partial replacements in 1991, the latest data available from the American Association of Orthopaedic Surgeons.

ETIOLOGIES

- Osteoarthritis with loss of joint cartilage
- Posttraumatic degeneration of joint structures
- Rheumatoid arthritis with or without avascular necrosis

CLINICAL MANIFESTATIONS

- Atrophy of deltoid muscles
- Deformity of shoulder joint
- Frequent subluxation or dislocation of the humeral head
- Pain with use of arm, when raising arm, and at rest

DIAGNOSTIC/CLINICAL FINDINGS

- History of falling on shoulder during sports games (especially football) with tear of rotator cuff tendons
- Physical examination revealing deformity of shoulder joint, atrophy of deltoid muscle, and pain on palpation of glenohumeral joint and acromiohumeral area (joint laxity)
- Positive apprehension and drop arm tests
- Roentgenograms computerized tomography (CT) and magnetic resonance imaging (MRI) showing osteophytes, loss of joint cartilage, some pannus, bone cysts, and loss of joint congruity

- Serologic studies revealing a positive rheumatoid factor, anemia (hemoglobin 11 g, hematocrit 30%) and white blood count (WBC) count of 6,700

▶ NURSING DIAGNOSIS: *Impaired Physical Mobility*

Related To anesthesia, shoulder replacement, and presence of orthosis (similar to an airplane splint)

Defining Characteristics

- Groggy from general anesthesia and muscle relaxant medication during surgery
- Moaning, wincing at times
- Orthosis restraining operative arm, elbow, and forearm

Patient Outcomes

The patient will

- be able to abduct operative shoulder to 90° in 7–10 days postoperatively.
- be ambulatory on first postoperative day with orthosis on operative arm.
- begin internal rotation of operative arm after third postoperative week with permission.
- begin passive, then active, exercises of wrist/hand, elbow, and finally operative shoulder as prescribed.

Nursing Interventions	Rationales
Assess operative arm from shoulder to fingers, noting dressing, drainage, position of arm, and security of orthosis.	Operative arm should be abducted with neutral rotation [some physicians use an abduction pillow or modified Dunlop's skin traction in place of an orthotic device; the arm may also be placed in a continuous passive motion (CPM) machine]. The dressing should cover the anterior incision, and there may be drainage present from wound drains. The pressure-sensitive straps should hold the arm securely. The patient should be able to move fingers and wrist actively.
Position patient on back to maintain operative arm in the required abducted position.	The arm is abducted to help maintain the prosthetic humeral head in the glenoid fossa. Newer prostheses may be noncemented, press fit into

Nursing Interventions	Rationales
	the humeral shaft, with modular, removable humeral "head" prostheses. The glenoid prosthesis may be cemented and held with screws. A bone graft may be used (particularly in persons with rheumatoid arthritis who have poor bone stock) to build up the glenoid area for more secure replacement.
Massage shoulder, neck, and back areas q3–4h.	Because of the position in bed, the mentioned areas become tight and tense. Massage loosens the muscles and helps relaxation.
When permitted, assist the patient to sit on the bedside, then in a chair, then to ambulate. Be sure an airplane splint or the orthosis is in place.	Ambulation helps maintain muscle/joint strength and helps the patient develop a positive outlook toward recovery.
Seek consultation with physical therapists for exercise protocol: passive (via a CPM machine) and active exercises are begun according to physician's prescription.	Passive exercises are done to maintain some functions. Active exercises are begun on the first postoperative day, as permitted, to help the operative arm regain functions. Limitations include no internal rotation for 3 or more weeks postoperatively to avoid the possibility of joint disruption.

NOTE: The remainder of the nursing diagnoses after total shoulder are very similar to those following a total hip and will not be repeated to avoid redundancy.

DISCHARGE PLANNING/CONTINUITY OF CARE

- Refer to physical therapy for long-term rehabilitation exercise regimen.
- Refer to home care nurses for wound care and assistance with activities of daily living as needed.
- Secure follow-up physician's appointment.
- Provide written instructions for medication regimen, their purposes, and side effects.

REFERENCES

Craig, E. V. (1988). Total shoulder replacement: Indications and results. *Orthopedics, 11*(1), 125–140.

Dines, D. M. (Chair, Round Table), Bigliani, L. U., Cofield, R. H., Hawkins, R. J., & Warren, R. F. (1992). Shoulder arthroplasty. *Orthopedic Special Edition, 1*(2), 1, 6–21.

Ellman, H. (1988). Shoulder arthroscopy: Current indications and techniques. *Orthopedics, 11*(1), 45–52.

Fu, F. H. (Moderator), Burkhead, W. Z. Jr., Flatow, E. L., Gerber, C., Harryman, D. T., II., Johnson, L. L., O'Driscoll, S., Perry, J., Snyder, S. J., & Warner, J. P. (1993). Symposium: Controversies in reconstruction of the unstable shoulder: Mobility versus instability—Part II. *Contemporary Orthopaedics, 26*(4), 407–427.

Johnson, R. L. (1993). Total shoulder arthroplasty. *Orthopaedic Nursing, 12*(1), 14–22.

Peterson, C. A., & Newton, S. E., III. (1991). Arthroscopic Bankart repair. *American Journal of Arthroscopy, 1*(2), 17–19.

Rounseville, C. (1992). Phantom limb pain: The ghost that haunts the amputee. *Orthopaedic Nursing, 11*(2), 67–71.

Varmarken, J. E., & Jensen, C. H. (1989). Recurrent anterior dislocation of the shoulder: Comparison of results after the Bankart and Putti-Platt procedures. *Orthopaedic Review, 12*(3), 453–456.

Other Surgical Procedures

Along with the previously mentioned surgeries, there are other orthopaedic surgical interventions, including amputation, replantation of amputated tissues, ligament and cartilage repairs, and limb-lengthening procedures.

Although antibiotics and microsurgical and limb-salvage techniques have made amputation less-common, this procedure is sometimes still necessary. Patients undergoing an amputation require the sensitive, supportive care of all health team members to assist the patient and family in working through the grieving process and developing a realistic outlook for the future.

With the advent of microsurgical techniques and instrumentation, severed or amputated limbs, digits, and toes may, at times, be reattached to the remaining tissues. Amputated parts may be completely severed or incompletely severed, being still attached by skin or other tissues. Reattaching the severed part(s) is called replantation.

A part or parts may be severed by a clean cut, referred to as a guillotine amputation. Two other ways parts are severed are crush injuries, usually with much soft tissue damage, and avulsion injuries, which frequently are incomplete amputations, with skin degloving and marked soft tissue damage.

Replantation of an amputated part is dependent upon how long it has been since the injury and the care of the amputated part, as successful replantation must be done before 12 h if warm ischemia has transpired.

Also, if there are large amounts of muscle and nerve tissue damage, replantation success is unpredictable, because of marked muscle ischemia.

The amputated part(s) must be carefully handled from the period of the initial injury to the time of replantation. The part(s) should be wrapped in a clean, dry, cool cloth and moistened with normal saline or Ringer's lactate solution, if available from emergency medical personnel. If these solutions are not available, the parts should be wrapped and placed in a sealed plastic bag and then the bag should be placed in ice water. If the amputation was incomplete, the partially loose parts should be packed in a moist sponge on ice (Higgins, 1991).

The rotator cuff, consisting of the muscles and tendons surrounding the shoulder joint, provides strength and stability to the shoulder joint. Repetitive stress, such as the overhead throwing actions of athletes, and degenerative or traumatic conditions of less-active persons can lead to impingement of one or more ligaments or tendons of the joint. Impingement causes pain, thus limiting the person's ability and desire to continue repetitive functions. Ultrasonography and arthroscopic examination of the shoulder, changes in operative positioning for optimal visibility, and use of rehabilitative exercises with a gradual return to previous activities, have made these repairs more lasting and often enable return to pre-trauma range of motion.

The cartilage (meniscus) pads of the knee can be damaged by a fall or a blow or twist of the knee. Aging can also cause damage to the meniscus. Recent use of less-invasive arthroscopic examination and repairs of these injuries has radically changed the care of patients with knee conditions. Research has shown that meniscal regeneration occurs, so that less meniscal tissue may need to be removed. Also, meniscal shaving, suturing, or laser repairs can be successfully done, resulting in a quicker return to usual activities for the patient. Meniscal injuries may be associated with knee ligament injuries, which may require arthroscopic/arthrotomy treatment.

Limb-lengthening techniques were developed in the Soviet Union by Dr. Gavriil Ilizarov, who performed a cutting (osteotomy) of the cortex (corticotomy) of the affected bone. The corticotomy did not damage the bone marrow, and the limb was then placed in a specially designed external fixator to allow the bone to heal and new bone to be laid in the osteomotized area. Through planned, timed adjustments (distractions) of the fixator, the limb was gradually lengthened, and the bone healed because circulation through the periosteum and endosteum brought about regeneration of the bone in the corticotomy gap. The Ilizarov technique can be used to correct bone, joint, or soft tissue conditions.

AMPUTATION

Amputation involves removal of part or all of one or more fingers, forearms, arms, thighs, legs, feet, or toes. Orthopaedically the lower limbs are amputated more frequently than other limbs, fingers, or toes, related to the more frequent occurrence of bone tumors, traumatic tissue and bone damage, circulatory inadequacies, or infection such as osteomyelitis.

ETIOLOGIES

- Crush injury to leg and foot
- Malignant bone tumor of distal femur
- Recalcitrant (not responding to treatments), chronic, multifocal osteomyelitis

CLINICAL MANIFESTATIONS

- Multiple open fractures of knee, tibia/fibula, with much soft tissue damage and loss
- Osteomyelitis, chronic, multiple open lesions
- Osteosarcoma of distal femur

DIAGNOSTIC/CLINICAL FINDINGS

- Chest roentgenogram negative for tumor metastases
- Magnetic resonance imaging (MRI) showing vascularity of tumor and presence of mass
- Physical examination revealing large mass in distal femur
- Roentgenograms of distal femur showing sunburst appearance characteristic of osteosarcoma
- Alkaline phosphatase level elevated in serum if a bone tumor is present
- Draining purulent material from multiple openings on leg, if osteomyelitis is present
- Roentgenograms showing presence of sequestrum in one site

▶ NURSING DIAGNOSIS: *Impaired Physical Mobility*

Related To above-knee amputation (AKA)

Defining Characteristics

- Postoperative diagnosis of chronic osteomyelitis
- Presence of AKA

Patient Outcomes

The patient will

- experience no recurrence of osteomyelitis.
- regain physical mobility, initially with crutches, then with prosthesis for ambulation.

Nursing Interventions	Rationales
Assess stump dressing for drainage, edema, and position of stump.	Wound may have serosanguineous drainage from operative site on dressing. The stump may have mild edema. The stump should be elevated on one pillow for 24 h. The stump should be held in neutral position (not abducted or adducted).
Clarify purposes of elevation of stump for only 24 h.	It is elevated only for 24 h to lessen edema formation and is then placed flat to prevent development of contractures.
Reposition or turn patient q4h.	Turning increases circulation and lessens pressure on bony prominences.
Seek consultation with physical therapists to teach proper exercises and crutch-walking techniques.	Exercises will include thigh adduction to help prevent abduction contractures plus stump extension exercises to prevent flexion contractures of stump. Initially, the patient will use a walker or crutches to ambulate until stump has healed and is properly shaped for fitting into the prosthesis.
Assist patient to ambulate with crutches.	The patient will feel “unbalanced” without the rest of the lower limb. Assistance is necessary for safety and

Nursing Interventions	Rationales
	security until patient feels more secure with crutches or walker.
Encourage range-of-motion (ROM) exercise to unaffected joints.	Range-of-motion exercises help patient maintain strength in muscles/joints.
Assist orthotist with measuring patient for prosthesis.	Measurements are taken so prosthesis may be made for use when stump area is ready for fitting.

▶ NURSING DIAGNOSIS: *Body Image Disturbance*

Related To loss of limb

Defining Characteristics

- Above-knee amputation of lower limb
- Patient is quiet, reserved, and hesitant to leave room

Patient Outcomes

The patient will

- become more comfortable in social setting and interactions.
- regain a positive body image.

Nursing Interventions	Rationales
Assess patient's reactions and responses to amputation.	Patient may not be able to verbalize or voice concerns in early postoperative period, but only when he or she feels more comfortable with nursing personnel.
Introduce patient to health team members and other patients, if appropriate.	Introductions may help patient feel less isolated.
Listen to patient when able to voice concerns; allow sufficient time to have clear understanding of concerns.	Intimate (personal) conversations take time to be expressed, and clarifications are often needed for clear understandings.
Seek consultation with social service, if needed.	Social services may assist patient with solutions to financial or other concerns.

Nursing Interventions	Rationales
If patient agrees, have a person wearing an above-knee prosthesis visit.	Seeing and talking with a person with an amputation to learn of problems or challenges should help the patient adjust to these same situations as they arise.
Encourage the patient to wear own clothing and to meet and interact with other patients.	Wearing own clothing helps the person become more positive and outward looking.
Reiterate patient's advances in use of crutches for going up and down stairs.	Praising patient helps patient realize progress is being noticed and made.

▶ NURSING DIAGNOSIS: *High Risk for Injury*

Risk Factors

- Above-knee amputation for chronic osteomyelitis
- Operative wound closed with skin sutures/clips with penrose drain in one end of incision

Patient Outcomes

The patient will

- experience wound healing by first intention.
- have no arterial bleeding.
- not develop a wound infection.

Nursing Interventions	Rationales
Assess stump incisional area for signs of wound healing, including presence of redness, edema, increased amount or type of drainage, and appearance of skin clips or sutures.	Redness and edema should markedly lessen by postoperative day 3 or 4. Drainage should also become serous and slight after initially being sanguineous and serosanguineous and moderate in amount. There should be "sealing" with beginning collagen in incisional area with no gaps or openings except at penrose drain site. The penrose drain may be removed on postoperative day 3 or 4.

Nursing Interventions	Rationales
Have a tourniquet present on bedside stand.	A tourniquet may be applied to the stump area if there is a large or moderate amount of bright red bleeding, which may signify opening of an artery. If the bleeding does not stop, the patient may need resuturing to stop the bleeding. If used, the tourniquet should only be applied tight enough to stop the bleeding and should be loosened to allow cellular perfusion.
Monitor vital signs q4h for first 24 h postopertively, then as usual, if temperature not elevated.	Frequent checks of vital signs and temperatures help detect abnormalities early so attention can be given to offset any pathogens before an infection develops in the wound or elsewhere in the body. Elevations in body temperature above 100 F (37.8 C) and pulse rates above 100 beats/min should be reported to the physician if after the first postoperative day.
Change wound dressings using aseptic technique.	Cleaning wound/incision and changing dressings frequently decrease chance of an infection developing.
Administer antibiotics as prescribed.	Antibiotics help prevent infections.
Teach patient/family members stump-wrapping techniques and wound care as appropriate.	Stump wrapping is done to shape the stump so it will fit snugly into the top of the prosthesis so pressure is decreased on the incisional area.

▶ NURSING DIAGNOSIS: *Acute Pain*

Related To surgical incision and nerve severing

Defining Characteristics

- Preoperative pain in areas of osteomyelitis
- Presence of incisional area in midthigh

Patient Outcomes

The patient will

- be relieved of painful episodes with prescribed medications.
- not experience phantom pain.

Nursing Interventions	Rationales
Assess complaints of pain [if patient-controlled analgesia (PCA) pump not in use]; its type, severity, duration; and patient's efforts to relieve pain.	Acute pain is expected after surgical amputation because of interruption of nerve transmissions and pressure on nerve endings. Phantom pain is the sensation of burning, tingling, pressure, and aching or itching in the stump area as if the amputated part is still present. It may be related to the preoperative pathology or to the surgical trauma and may last or linger for several months or longer after amputation.
Reposition and turn patient q2–4h; turn to abdomen q4h.	Repositioning increases circulation to remove wastes and relieve pain or discomfort. Turning to abdomen extends thigh to relax muscles and helps prevent flexion contractures as well as relieves discomfort or pain.
Administer analgesic medications q4h if PCA pump not in use; if so, monitor amount of analgesic needed to relieve pain.	Analgesics relieve pain through their central nervous system actions so pain is not felt. A PCA pump helps the patient feel more in control as he or she can self-administer analgesic according to preset amounts and times. It helps patients feel more independent.
Clarify gradual regression of phantom pain over time.	As surgical trauma and preoperative pathology are relieved, the severity and appearance of phantom pain gradually decrease until the episodes are no longer of concern. Persistent phantom pain must be investigated by the physician to determine its cause.

DISCHARGE PLANNING/CONTINUITY OF CARE

- Refer to home care nurses for stump wrapping techniques and wound care and assistance with activities of daily living as needed.
- Refer to physical therapy for extension exercises and ambulation assistance.
- Refer to orthotist for follow-up visits for prosthetic fittings.
- Secure follow-up physician's appointment.

REFERENCES

Anderson, M. A., & Helms, L. (1993). An assessment of discharge planning models: Communication in referrals for home care. *Orthopaedic Nursing, 12*(4), 41–48.

Lewis, S. M., & Collier, I. C. (1992). *Medical-surgical nursing.* St. Louis: Mosby-Yearbook.

Mourad, L. A. (1991). *Orthopedic disorders.* St. Louis: Mosby-Yearbook.

Rounseville, C. (1992). Phantom limb pain: The ghost that haunts the amputee. *Orthopaedic Nursing, 11*(2), 67–71.

Williamson, V. C. (1992). Amputation of the lower extremity: An overview. *Orthopaedic Nursing, 11*(2), 55–65.

REPLANTATION OF AMPUTATED PARTS

ETIOLOGIES

- Complete or incomplete amputation of a part or limb
- Presence of minimal soft tissue damage by a guillotine amputation of dominant hand/forearm

CLINICAL MANIFESTATIONS

- Hand severed from forearm 2 in. above wrist
- Hand wrapped and placed in plastic bag placed in ice water
- Remaining forearm tissues wrapped with clean bandages with bright red blood saturation

CLINICAL/DIAGNOSTIC FINDINGS

- History of using a power saw to cut logs. Hand amputated as patient grabbed a dog to prevent injury to the dog after it jumped on a log. Patient is a 22-year-old male farm worker.
- Physical examination reveals a clean, guillotine cut of forearm, with amputated hand present in bag/ice water.
- Roentgenograms reveal no fractures of proximal radius or ulna, but tearing of radioulnar ligament. No fractures of distal portions of radius and ulna are present in the hand portion. Patient is very alert and anxious.
- Laboratory tests reveal hemoglobin of 13.2 g/100 mL and hematocrit of 33%. Platelet count is 210,000.

▶ NURSING DIAGNOSIS: *Anxiety*

Related To sudden trauma and amputation 1 h prior to admission

Defining Characteristics

- Has marked restlessness, moaning, and turning legs side to side on gurney almost constantly
- Holding onto right forearm with lift hand; seems to be protecting right forearm; does not want personnel to touch area
- Skin of face and neck covered with perspiration; clothes (shirt) wet with apparent perspiration and blood
- Color of exposed skin areas very pale and cool
- Is very alert, eyes darting around from health team member to member, repeatedly looking at all equipment in room

Patient Outcomes

The patient will

- experience lower levels of anxiety over time.
- have less restlessness, nervousness, and perspiration.
- permit health team members to handle affected parts and to provide definitive care.

Nursing Interventions	Rationales
Assess level of anxiety: observe alertness, moaning, turning side to side, and hesitance to let go of remaining forearm tissues.	Observations help determine appropriate interventions to help decrease the patient's anxiety.
Talk to and reassure patient while proceeding with admission procedures and assessments.	Speaking calmly and clearly helps the patient refocus on situation and care.
Explain upcoming events or clarify physician's explanations.	Anxiety may prevent patient's continued attention to physician's explanations, and clarification may be required more than once. Explanations lessen anxiety.
Assist with physical examination and diagnostic tests; explain while participating.	Assistance permits examination and testing to be completed expeditiously, thereby lessening patient disturbance.
Do preoperative preparation.	Replantation is begun as soon as possible because of need to reestablish circulation to the amputated part.

Nursing Interventions	Rationales
Allow family/significant others to stay with patient until surgery.	Anxiety is reduced by having family/significant others close to patient.
Monitor vital signs and intravenous therapy.	Patient may have hypovolemic shock from hemorrhage after amputation, reflected in lower blood pressure and rapid pulse.

▶ NURSING DIAGNOSIS: *High Risk for Additional Injury (Circulatory Compromise)*

Risk Factors

- Repair of small arteries
- Repair of at least one vein
- Insufficient elevation
- Proximity to wrist making circulatory repairs more tenuous for regaining full circulation

Patient Outcomes

The patient will

- regain adequate arterial inflow.
- regain satisfactory venous return.
- have mild edema only.
- experience no arterial clotting or phlebitis.

Nursing Interventions	Rationales
Assess circulatory status hourly: color, capillary refill, temperature, turgor, and edema.	Circulatory checks should be done under the same lighting conditions for most accurate comparisons. New-shift personnel should compare their findings with personnel who have been doing the hourly assessments for accuracy.
Report loss of arterial pulses or venous stasis [noted by capillary refill that is too fast (1–2 s) and marked edema].	Loss of circulation and circulatory compromise are emergencies and should be reported promptly. The patient will possibly return to surgery for examination and correction.

Nursing Interventions	**Rationales**
Assist with loosening tight dressings, if required.	Loosening too-tight dressings may allow circulation to be regained without surgical exploration.
Lower elevation of limb to heart level.	Lowering limb to heart level allows arterial inflow without compromising venous return.
Apply medicinal leeches to digits as prescribed.	Leeches (Hirudo medicinalis) ingest 30–50 mL of blood each to lessen congestion and promote bleeding. Venous congestion and edema are lessened and venous return is fostered. Each leech will attach itself to a bleeding puncture wound and drop off when satiated (20–30 min). Three to five or more leeches may be used.
Destroy the used leeches by placing in a solution of alcohol or saline and seal the container.	The leeches will die in these solutions. Dispose of the container with other biohazardous waste (Higgins, 1991).
Monitor oxygen content in digits with pulse oximeter.	Pulse oximeters provide continuous recordings of oxygen saturation content in arteries in digits. Readings of 94–100% are within normal limits (WNL).
Monitor perfusion of replanted digits by Doppler or use of fluorescein dye.	Doppler monitoring provides data of red blood cell (RBC) movements via an implanted crystal in the reattached artery. Arterial flow is noted by a pulsing sound, and venous flow is noted by a "whooshing" sound (Higgins, 1991). Fluorescence under ultraviolet light indicates perfusion at the reanastomosis site.
Monitor local and systemic temperatures.	Infection in the replanted or amputated parts is a possibility if the initial injury was not sterile or clean or it may develop from the leech therapy.

Nursing Interventions	Rationales
Administer broad-spectrum antibiotics as prescribed.	Organisms usually respond to the use of cephalosporins or aminoglysides given q6h for 5–7 days.
Administer aspirin daily and Persantine t.i.d. as prescribed.	Aspirin and Persantine inhibit plalelet aggregation to decrease clot formation. Persantine also dilates peripheral small arteries.
Administer heparin subcutaneously as prescribed.	Heparin dosage is dependent on results of partial thromboplastin (PTT) test (desired range is one and a half to two times normal PTT of patient. Heparin inhibits clot formation.
Administer nifedipine as prescribed.	Nifedipine acts as a peripheral vasodilator and also inhibits platelet aggregation. It is given for 7–10 days postoperatively.
Prevent any smoking by personnel caring for patient, relatives, or visitors.	Smoking constricts peripheral vessels and is contraindicated by everyone coming in contact with the patient.

▶ NURSING DIAGNOSIS: *Impaired Physical Mobility*

Related To prescribed bedrest and nonfunctional limb

Defining Characteristics

- Bedrest for 4–5 days
- Motor functions of replanted tissues not immediately functioning postoperatively

Patient Outcomes

The patient will

- have successful replantation after long-term recovery.
- become ambulatory when permitted.
- maintain operative arm in immobilizer and sling, if prescribed.

Nursing Interventions	Rationales
Assess bony prominences twice daily for redness, whiteness, or open lesions.	Bedrest may cause pressure on bony prominences, leading to circulatory compromise and formation of decubiti.
Massage back and around bony prominences twice daily.	Massage increases circulation, lessens tight muscles, and increases sense of well-being and relaxation.
Reposition patient q2–3h.	Changing positions aids relaxation and lessens pressure on bony prominences.
Consult with physical and occupational therapists for prescribed exercise and splinting regimens.	Passive exercises are begun approximately 1 week postoperatively. Active exercises may be started after second postoperative week. Splints are used to maintain desired positions of replanted hand and digits. An external fixator may be used to immobilize radius and ulna for bone healing.
Secure consult for social services.	Social services assist with long-term financial, psychologic, and employment needs of the patient and family.

▶ NURSING DIAGNOSIS: *Knowledge Deficit*

Related To unfamiliarity with present and future events

Defining Characteristics

- Unfamiliarity with terms microsurgery, replantation, circulation checks, and passive and active exercises
- Presence of anxiety and shock
- Lack of certainty about outcome

Patient Outcomes

The patient will

- understand explanations of surgical repairs and replantation.
- accept over time the uncertainty of long-term results.
- have lower level of anxiety about surgery and postoperative care.
- regain physiologic equilibrium after treatments for shock.

Nursing Interventions	Rationales
Assess knowledge and understanding following physician's explanations by asking pertinent questions.	Patient's answers give evidence of understanding.
Clarify partial or unclear information as needed.	Patient's anxiety and shock states may preclude full attention and/or understanding.
Repeat schedule of immediate and intraoperative events.	Repetition is needed due to unfamiliar and emergency situation.
Allow patient/family/significant others to ask questions.	These people may be able to ask vital questions that may not occur to patient because of condition or diagnostic examinations.
Provide realistic encouragement to patient and concerned others.	The nurse's previous experiences and knowledge of upcoming care and recovery stages or patterns are beneficial and positive.
Provide patient/relatives/significant others with ongoing or updated information as postoperative course proceeds.	Maintaining progressive communications is reassuring over time.
Teach self-care as needed to patient and home caregivers.	Learning self-care lessens concerns of ability to care for needs after discharge.

DISCHARGE PLANNING/CONTINUITY OF CARE

- Complete referral to home care nurses to monitor wound healing, exercise regimen, and nutritional needs as warranted.
- Refer to occupational therapists for specific exercises and splints required.
- Refer to social services for ongoing psychologic, financial, or employment needs.
- Secure appointment for follow-up visit to physician.

REFERENCES

Casady, L., & Scaduto, J. (1991). Thumb replantation: A case study. *Orthopaedic Nursing, 10*(3), 24.

Higgins, R. M. (1991). Replantation of digits. *Orthopaedic Nursing, 10*(3), 11–18.

Iglesias, M., & Serano, A. (1990). Replantation of amputated segments after prolonged ischemia. *Plastic and Reconstructive Surgery, 85*(3), 425–479.

Ramasastry, S. (1990). Replantation. *Trauma Rounds, 2*(3).

ROTATOR CUFF REPAIRS

The rotator cuff surrounds the shoulder joint. It is made up of muscles and their tendons which hold the humeral head in the glenoid. The cuff is comprised of the supraspinatus, teres minor, and infraspinatus muscles, which rotate the humerus externally, and the subscapularis, which rotates the humerus internally. These muscles, plus the deltoid, provide stability to the shoulder joint. Instability and tears are two conditions necessitating repairs of the rotator cuff (see Table 24.1, page 241).

ETIOLOGIES

- Complete anterior or posterior dislocation of humeral head
- Congenital anomalies such as abnormal tilt to glenoid soft tissue laxity or neurologic disorders
- Direct or indirect trauma to tendons or muscles
- Overuse activities, most often sports related
- Partial or complete tears of one or more tendons of rotator cuff muscles
- Repetitive employment-related stressful movements of shoulders
- Subluxation (partial dislocation) of humeral head from glenoid

CLINICAL MANIFESTATIONS

- Apprehension and fear that some movements will cause subluxation or dislocation
- Decreased range-of-motion (ROM) of shoulder joint
- Feeling that arm has "gone dead"
- History of occupational or sports activities requiring lifting and overhead movements
- Muscle(s) atrophy, such as the deltoid
- Night pain that may radiate down arm to elbow
- Shoulder instability
- Tenderness around glenoid and humeral head

CLINICAL/DIAGNOSTIC FINDINGS

- Arthrogram shows dye in tear area

- Arthroscopy shows tear in tendons and tears in the glenoid labrum
- Decreased ROM of joint and complaint of temporary numbness
- Electromyogram may show nerve dysfunction
- Pain and tenderness on palpation
- Physical examination elicits shoulder instability with or without reproducible subluxation or dislocation of humeral head, muscle/soft tissue laxity, muscle atrophy; examination of the neck must be done to determine if cervical pathology is causing the shoulder pain
- Roentgenograms may show degenerative changes, partial subluxation
- Ultrasound or magnetic resonance imaging (MRI) will show tear in one or more cuff tendons

▶ NURSING DIAGNOSIS: *Impaired Physical Mobility (Preoperatively)*

Related To tear of rotator cuff tendons and instability of shoulder joint

Defining Characteristics

(As given under Clinical Manifestations)

Patient Outcomes

The patient will

- regain a more stable shoulder joint after treatments.
- undergo conservative treatment for 3 or more weeks.
- undergo long-term rehabilitation for 9–12 months .
- undergo surgical repair if conservative treatment fails to relieve pain or prevent recurring instability.

Nursing Interventions	Rationales
Assess shoulder ROM (can use physician's examination findings to avoid causing additional pain) and site of pain or tenderness and discuss when pain occurs, if with use.	Assessment data provide the basis for individual's treatment protocol.
Apply sling to affected arm with arm in internal rotation.	Placing arm in sling provides rest to the joint to avoid continuing irritation to the tissues.
Apply cold therapy for 15 min three times daily for 3 days.	Cold causes vasoconstriction to decrease edema, if present, and to decrease pain.

Nursing Interventions	Rationales
Administer prescribed analgesics and anti-inflammatories.	Analgesics relieve pain; anti-inflammatory medications decrease inflammation.
Secure consultation with physical therapy for prescribed exercises.	Gentle ROM exercises are done after about 3 weeks of rest in the sling to decrease or prevent adhesions and other complications of immobility.
Instruct patient of need to continue exercise program and to alternate applications of heat and cold after exercising.	Conservative treatments of exercises, heat, and cold will be continued for 9–12 months to strengthen shoulder to increase stability and relieve pain. If the patient is young, he or she may experience recurrence of symptoms as they are more active than older persons, who are less likely to put themselves at risk.

▶ NURSING DIAGNOSIS: *Impaired Physical Mobility (Postoperatively)*

Related To anesthesia or surgical procedure

Defining Characteristics

- Bankart or Bristow repair (see descriptions, page 243) or other corrective repair
- General anesthesia for shoulder repair

Patient Outcomes

The patient will

- be able to return to usual activities after rehabilitation.
- be relieved of recurring dislocations and pain.
- regain ROM of operative shoulder after exercise program and rehabilitation.

Nursing Interventions	Rationales
Assess operative arm for presence of sling and swathe or orthosis, dressing over incision, presence of drain, and drainage and edema.	The operative arm will be held in a sling or orthosis to maintain the integrity of the operative repair until the muscles and tendons have healed sufficiently to hold the humeral head in the glenoid. The incision will be anterior most often.
Reposition the patient q2–3h.	Repositioning relaxes tired muscles and increases circulation to remove wastes.
Encourage deep breathing and use of incentive spirometer.	Deep breathing helps oxygenate all lung areas. The incentive spirometer adds deep inhalation and lung expansion to enhance oxygenation.
Assist patient to ambulate with operative arm in sling and swathe or orthosis.	Because both arms can not swing freely, the patient may feel unbalanced; therefore, assistance is needed for safety and security.
Secure consultation with physical therapy to begin passive, then active, exercises as prescribed.	Physical therapists begin to assist the patient with the exercise regimen required over 1 year so the patient can regain the strength in the muscles. Passive exercises are done with active exercises and gradual weight lifting not starting for 3 months for some patients.
Teach patient/family members how to apply the sling and swathe or the orthosis.	Knowing how to apply these devices increases the patient's independence and self-confidence.

NOTE: Other nursing diagnoses for rotator cuff repairs are similar to those for total shoulder replacement and will not be repeated here to avoid redundancy.

Table 24.1 • Surgical Treatments for Rotator Cuff Injuries

Bankart repair	Involves suturing the labrum and capsule to the glenoid rim and repair of any tears in supraspinatus tendon, if present
Bristow repair	Involves repair of the glenoid labrum and joint capsule with an anterior bone block attached with a screw to add stability to the repair and capsule shift
Capsulorrhaphy	Repair of the shoulder capsule ligaments and tendon attachments
Wedge osteotomy	A wedge of bone may be taken from the outer surface of the humerus to change the angle of the head of the humerus in the glenoid to decrease subluxation and/or dislocation
Posterior capsule shift or anterior-inferior capsule shift	Joint capsule ligaments and tendons are cut and resewn laterally and distally (the superior flap; the inferior flap is advanced laterally and proximally); the goal of surgery is to restore normal anatomic structures to prevent recurrence of instability and tears

DISCHARGE PLANNING/CONTINUITY OF CARE

- Refer to home care nurses for wound care and assistance with activities of daily living as needed.
- Refer to physical therapy for rehabilitation regimen and exercises.
- Secure follow-up appointment with physician.
- Provide written instructions for medication regimen, their purposes, and expected side effects.

REFERENCES

Brems, J. (1988). Rotator cuff tear: Evaluation and treatment. *Orthopaedic Review, 18*(3), 364–375.

Morrison, D. S., & Ofstein, R. (1990). The use of magnetic resonance imaging in the diagnosis of rotator cuff tears. *Orthopedics, 13*(6), 633–637.

Seitz, W. H., Froimson, A. I., & Shapiro, J. D. (1989). Chronic impingement syndrome. *Orthopaedic Review, 18*(3), 364–375.

Worland, R. L. (1993). Treatment of rotator cuff impingement. *Orthopaedic Review, 22*(I), 76–79.

MENISCAL REPAIRS

The menisci are the crescent-shaped cartilage pads attached to the top of the tibia within the knee joint. The menisci are major weight-bearing structures, taking more than half of the load transmitted across the joint. They are "fillers" between the femoral and tibial surfaces which help enhance the surface lubrication of the joint. They also provide some rotary stability to the knee joint.

Tears can occur in the menisci at the ends (anterior or posterior third areas), in the middle third, or longitudinally, the so-called bucket-handle tear. Because of blood supply and vascularization, tears in the outer fourth of the meniscus will heal; however, tears in the inner, avascular area will not heal. The medial meniscus (inner side of knee) is torn three times more frequently than the lateral one.

ETIOLOGIES

- Athletic (sports related) or occupational (e.g., miners, roofers, and others) injury
- Rotational movements of the tibia on femur with the knee partially flexed or extended
- Squatting with the knee acutely flexed; tearing when twisting and rising from the squatting position
- Varus or valgus thrust or movements may trap and tear the meniscus
- Associated tears of medial or lateral capsular ligaments

CLINICAL MANIFESTATIONS

- Acute pain on inner or outer surface of the knee
- History of injury and repeated knee locking unexpectedly
- Inability to straighten the knee and leg
- "Locking" of knee without warning
- Marked tenderness of knee
- Rapid swelling of knee

CLINICAL/DIAGNOSTIC FINDINGS

- Arthrography: may or may not reveal tear or tears
- Arthroscopy: will reveal tears if joint fluid is clear enough
- Physical examination shows marked effusion (swelling) of knee joint line, with pain produced if knee is put in forced adduction, and person may be unable to fully flex knee
- Positive McMurray sign: patient's tibia held in external rotation and abduction and knee slowly extended from fully flexed position; a click felt at the posterior joint line if there is a posterior tear in the medial meniscus; for lateral meniscus check, leg held with knee in flexion, adduction, and internal rotation
- Roentgenograms: may be negative for tears but done to rule out loose bodies, osteoarthritis, or fracture

▶ NURSING DIAGNOSIS: *Impaired Physical Mobility*

Related To one or more meniscal tears

Defining Characteristics

- Acute pain in knee
- Edema and joint effusion
- Inability to straighten knee to walk and bear weight
- Locking of knee

Patient Outcomes

The patient will

- be able to use knee joint normally after treatments.
- be able to return to usual employment and sports activities.
- regain a pain-free knee joint after treatments.
- retain full muscle strength while receiving treatments.

Nursing Interventions	Rationales
Assess knee area for edema, pain, motor and sensory functions, and position held by patient.	Data are helpful to determine pathology and for care plan.
Apply cold therapy to knee joint.	Cold constricts blood vessels to decrease bleeding and pain.
Assist with aspiration of knee joint, if done.	Aspiration of fluid provides data of nature of joint effusion. Bleeding may continue and reaspiration may need to be done.
Provide reassurance and support to patient if physician tries to reduce	Reduction may be attempted manually or with Buck traction.

Nursing Interventions	Rationales
the meniscal displacement (if knee is locked).	
Apply knee immobilizer splint after knee is extended.	The knee is held immobilized to permit healing of area, if possible. Usual time for knee extension is 3 weeks or until acute symptoms subside.
Encourage patient to begin quadriceps-setting exercises q4h and patella setting with the knee extended as prescribed.	Muscle-setting exercises maintain the muscle tone and strength. "Quad" setting is done by having the patient push the knee backward toward the bed while tightening the quadriceps muscle. When able, the patient sets the patella by tightening the quadriceps to feel the patella move.
Seek consultation with physical therapists for weight-lifting extension exercises when prescribed.	Weight-lifting exercises help strengthen muscles and restore normal mobility.
Clarify proposed surgical procedure to repair meniscal tear.	Surgical procedures usually are done arthroscopically during which the torn meniscus is removed, leaving intact or untorn meniscal cartilage in place. If the tear is in the vascular area of the meniscus, it may be sutured so it can heal.
Postoperatively, check position of knee immobilizer and wound dressing.	Immobilizer is used to prevent knee flexion. Wound dressing may be enclosing foot and leg up to midthigh.
Assist patient to be up with walker or crutches.	Ambulation is begun on first or second postoperative day.
Encourage patient to do quadriceps-setting and hamstring-strengthening exercises as prescribed.	Exercises help retain muscle strength.
Administer analgesic medications as prescribed.	Analgesics may be required for 1–3 days postoperatively.
Do all neurovascular checks q2h for 24 h, then q4h.	Neurovascular checks are vital because of possibility of thrombus formation from use of tourniquet during surgery.

Nursing Interventions	Rationales
Apply cold therapy to operative site.	Vasoconstriction lessens bleeding possibility.
Observe patient while doing straight-leg raises.	The patient usually must be able to raise leg to 60° elevation while keeping the knee straight prior to being discharged.
Obtain time and date for next patient visit to physician.	Having the next appointment time and date is reassuring to the patient.

DISCHARGE PLANNING/CONTINUITY OF CARE

- Provide written guidelines for neurovascular checks after discharge.
- Refer to physical therapy for leg-strengthening and straight-leg-raising exercises.
- Provide written medication regime, purposes, and expected side effects.
- Secure follow-up physician's appointment.

REFERENCES

DeHaven, K. E., Black, K. P., & Griffiths, H. J. (1989). Open meniscal repair: Technique and 2 to 9 year results. *American Journal of Sports Medicine, 17*(7), 788–795.

Diment, M. T., DeHaven, K. E., & Sebastianelli, W. J. (1993). Current concepts in meniscal repair. *Orthopedics, 16*(9), 973–977.

Hanks, G. A., Gause, T. M., Sebastianelli, W. J., O'Donnell, C. S., & Kalenak, A. (1991). Repair of peripheral meniscal tears: Open versus arthroscopic technique. *Arthroscopy, 7*(1), 72–77.

Hardin, G. T., Farr, J., Bach, B. R., Jr. (1993). Meniscal tears: Diagnosis, evaluation, and treatment. *Orthopaedic Review, 21*(11), 1311–1317.

LIMB-LENGTHENING PROCEDURES

Limb lengthening begins with an operation called a corticotomy, which is cutting the bone two-thirds to three-fourths of the circumference circularly through the cortex only, after the external fixator is applied. The fixator consists of "tensioned" (tightened) Kirschner wires attached to a series of full or half rings that encircle the affected limb. The wires may have an olive-shaped "stopper" on them, and these olive wires are used to achieve movement during the treatment (Newschwander & Dunst, 1989). By turning the two rings that lie on opposite sides of the corticotomy in opposite directions, the corticotomy is completed (Newschwander & Dunst, 1989). Postoperatively, the bone is distracted (pulled apart), beginning 2 or more days later, by turning the nuts a quarter turn every 6 h. In this method the cortex of the bone separates while the medullary canal and bone marrow and bone-forming cells continue to form new bone tissues as the distraction and lengthening proceed. Weight bearing is encouraged as part of the lengthening process.

Patient/family teaching in the use of the fixator is essential to ensuring successful adaptation.

ETIOLOGIES

- Fractured bone(s)
- Short limbs secondary to dwarfism or congenital or acquired deformity

CLINICAL MANIFESTATIONS

- Angular or rotational defect in one or more bones of limbs
- Inability to bear weight or use limb normally
- Presence of limp
- Psychologic concerns related to short stature

CLINICAL/DIAGNOSTIC FINDINGS

- History of achondroplasia, fracture, or defect in straightness or length of bone(s) of limb(s)
- Physical examination reveals shorter than normal stature and limbs or deformity of bone(s)
- Roentgenograms reveal normal bone mass but short length, deformity of bone(s), or fracture of bone(s)

▶ NURSING DIAGNOSIS: *Knowledge Deficit (Preoperative)*

Related To unfamiliar operative technique, external fixator and its purposes, and patient/family responsibilities

Defining Characteristics

- Concern for possible complications
- Fear of unknown
- No previous exposure or experience with external fixator(s), operation, or self-care to follow
- Unfamiliar terminology

Patient Outcomes

The patient will
- achieve bone healing (bone union) after corticotomy and lengthening procedures.
- experience no neurologic, circulatory, or wound complications.
- participate actively and positively in self-care.
- undergo limb lengthening with Ilizarov external fixator and corticotomy.

Nursing Interventions	Rationales
Assess patient/family's understandings after physician's explanations.	Newness of information may cause inattention or lack of complete understanding.
Clarify understanding, as appropriate, using a videotape or pictures of an Ilizarov external fixator (can have one applied to a doll).	Being able to see a picture or actual fixator placement should help the patient/family understand upcoming procedure and care more clearly.
Clarify possibility of patient's experiencing some drainage from operative and pin sites and having pain, along with care to deal with the drainage and pain.	Learning expected happenings helps patient accept them if or when they occur postoperatively as well as care to deal with them.

Nursing Interventions	Rationales
If available and agreed to by patient/family, have someone with a similar fixator visit the patient.	Seeing another person and being able to ask questions should ease patient's concerns.
Clarify required postapplication distraction procedure; allow patient/family members to do turning as required (on doll).	Practicing helps patient/family member become more comfortable with required care and provides the opportunity to observe interactions and performance of new skill.

▶ NURSING DIAGNOSIS: *Acute Pain (Postoperative)*

Related To unexpected discomfort and pain of cumbersome fixator

Defining Characteristics

- Complains of sharp pain around corticotomy site and pin sites
- Has fixator on humerus, radius/ulna, femur, or tibia
- Has patient-controlled analgesia (PCA) pump with morphine for narcotic analgesic

Patient Outcomes

The patient will

- have satisfactory relief of pain after administration of narcotic analgesia.
- regain comfort through use of play and visual or auditory distraction.

Nursing Interventions	Rationales
Assess complaints, severity, sites, and frequency of pain; assess wincing, crying, moaning, or other behaviors indicative of pain.	Pain experiences vary among individuals, but all behaviors should be responded to and medication should be given as prescribed.
Monitor effects of administration of narcotic analgesic or amount and use of PCA medication, if used.	Some patients have different pain tolerances, and adjustments may be required to aid patient's comfort.
Encourage patient to participate in play, games, or listening to music.	Diversionary techniques help distract the patient's attention to pain alone.
Administer narcotic analgesic orally, when prescribed.	Oral administration helps prevent fearfulness of injections and

Nursing Interventions	Rationales
	reassures patient that medication will not by itself inflict pain. Commonly used analgesics include age-titrated oxycodone or acetaminophen with codeine.

▶ NURSING DIAGNOSIS: *Impaired Physical Mobility*

Related To presence of fixator on femur, tibia, or humerus

Defining Characteristics

- Fixator in place on femur, tibia, or humerus
- Inability to bear weight without pain
- Initially, use of crutches or wheelchair if both lower limbs in fixators

Patient Outcomes

The patient will

- be able to gradually bear full weight as healing (union) proceeds.
- walk without crutches when permitted by healing.

Nursing Interventions	Rationales
Assess strength in arms to determine if can use crutches (or walker).	Patient must have enough strength and comfort to use crutches or walker for weight bearing until healing has progressed.
Seek consultation with physical therapists to assist with ambulation techniques.	Physical therapy is begun 3–4 days after corticotomy to assist with ambulation and strengthening exercises for crutch walking.
Check physical area for any obstructions to safe ambulation.	Patients may attempt to ambulate through areas too narrow to negotiate safely without hitting the fixator on furniture or walls. The area for patient's use should be free of sharp corners or immovable, heavy furniture for safety.
Observe patient's foot placement when walking.	Occasionally the patient may need a shoe orthosis for proper foot

Nursing Interventions	Rationales
	placement for optimal stepping and walking.

▶ NURSING DIAGNOSIS: *High Risk for Wound/Pin Site Infection*

Risk Factors

- Corticotomy around bone
- Multiple pin entrance sites
- Sanguineous drainage from pin insertion sites

Patient Outcomes

The patient will

- experience no wound or pin site infection.
- learn pin site care (or a family member will).

Nursing Interventions	Rationales
Assess all sites for presence and type of drainage.	Small amounts of sanguineous drainage are expected for 1–2 days after insertion of the pins.
Begin pin site care when prescribed.	Removal of drainage is needed to prevent skin maceration, drying or caking of sanguineous drainage, and possibility of infection. Site care involves moving the rubber stopper holding the dressing on the pin entrance site up away from the dressing and gently removing the old dressing. If secretions are dried, they can be loosened by dampening with hydrogen peroxide for ease in removing. Pin site care varies per physician, and no universally used protocol presently exists. Research has been unable to validate the effectiveness of selected pin site treatment modalities (Jones-Walton, 1991).

Nursing Interventions	Rationales
Clean each pin site of drainage, check for any signs of infection, replace the new dressing, and slide the rubber stopper down to hold it in place.	The stopper holds the sponge dressing and decreases skin movements at the pin sites to decrease the risk of infection and bleeding.
Observe all pin sites for marked redness or purulent drainage.	These are two signs of infection. Some edema of the operative limb is expected.
Elevate operative limb on a pillow.	Elevation increases venous return to lessen edema.
Observe patient/family member doing distraction technique.	Distraction is done using a 10-mm wrench. Specific printed instructions are placed at the bedside for use by all personnel. Instructions are specific to the type of rod being used in the external fixator, how much of a turn (one-fourth to one-half turn) and how many times a day the nut is to be turned.

DISCHARGE PLANNING/CONTINUITY OF CARE

- Provide written guidelines/instructions for distraction techniques; review carefully with patient/family/significant other.
- Refer to home care nurses for follow-up wound/pin site care and observing patient self-care.
- Refer to physical therapist for assistance with ambulation with crutches and range-of-motion exercises.
- Provide written information on medication regimen and purposes and expected side effects of medications.
- Secure follow-up physician's appointment.

REFERENCES

Elting, J. J., & Hubbell, J. C. (1993). Unilateral frame distraction: Proximal tibial valgus osteotomy for medial gonarthritis. *Contemporary Orthopaedics, 27*(5), 435–440.

Green, S. A. (1991). The Ilizarov method of orthopedic reconstruction. *Journal of Musculoskeletal Medicine, 8*(9), 83–96.

Jones-Walton, P. (1991). Clinical standards in skeletal traction pin site care. *Orthopaedic Nursing, 10*(2), 12–16.

Newschwander, G. E., & Dunst, R. M. (1989). Limb lengthening with the Ilizarov external fixator. *Orthopaedic Nursing, 8*(3), 15–21.

Sproul, J. T., & Price, C. T. (1992). Recent advances in limb lengthening. *Orthopaedic Review, 21*(4), 425–429.

Spinal Conditions

Various surgical procedures are done to repair or correct conditions involving the vertebral column. Such procedures include repair or removal of a herniated intervertebral disc; spinal fusion to correct deformities, fractures, or congenital anomalies; and insertion of intervertebral rods, screws, or plates to help maintain surgical corrections. The operations may be done percutaneously or through open surgical exposure. Patients may be discharged on the day of surgery or may be hospitalized for a week or longer, depending on the procedure and its outcome.

LAMINECTOMY OR PERCUTANEOUS DISCECTOMY

Either of the above operations may be done to remove herniated fragments of a herniated or ruptured disc. A laminectomy involves removal of part of the lamina to provide a route to the herniated disc particles for removal. A percutaneous discectomy is for patients who have not had previous back surgery, whose disc has ruptured posteriorly or laterally with no disc fragments in the spinal canal, or who are without lateral facet disease, lateral recess stenosis, or hypertrophy of the ligamentum flavum.

ETIOLOGIES

- Rupture of intervertebral disc with more than one fragment
- Degeneration of annulus (cartilage) around nucleus pulposus

CLINICAL MANIFESTATIONS

- History of low back pain with radiation down posterior side of one or both legs
- Complains of dull pain and pressure in lumbar area of back
- Complains of numbness of outer part of leg, lateral aspect of right foot, and outer three toes
- States it "hurts to try to stand up straight" or to stand up from a sitting position due to low back pain
- Unable to find a comfortable position in bed, which interferes with sleeping

CLINICAL/DIAGNOSTIC FINDINGS

- Physical examination reveals marked tenderness in lumbar and sacral areas of back
- Decreased ankle and Achilles reflexes

- Computerized tomography (CT) and magnetic resonance imaging (MRI) show multiple disc fragments protruding laterally and posteriorly from L_5 to S_1 disc space
- Hesitant to stand up from seated position because of pain in back
- Stands with "flat" back without normal lumbar lordosis
- Marked muscle tenseness in lower back

▶ NURSING DIAGNOSIS: *Acute Pain*

Related To herniated nucleus pulposus and pressure on spinal nerve

Defining Characteristics

- (See Clinical/Diagnostic Findings above)

Patient Outcomes

The patient will

- experience relief of back pain and nerve pressure after treatments.
- have no recurrence of back pain.
- be able to return to usual roles, responsibilities, and employment.

Nursing Interventions	Rationales
Assess site, severity, duration, and characteristics of patient's pain.	Patients vary in the site and severity of pain depending on which nucleus pulposus has herniated and in which direction it has herniated (e.g., laterally or posteriorly); also, pain may be of different types (burning, aching, persistent) depending on whether or not there is pressure on the spinal nerve at the site of herniation.
Place patient in prescribed rest and bed position.	Bedrest in Williams position with knees and head of bed elevated to 45° relax lumbosacral muscles optimally. Bedrest also decreases inflammation.
Administer prescribed medications q4h.	Medications may include narcotic analgesics, muscle relaxants and nonsteroidal anti-inflammatory medications.
Monitor effects of medications.	If pain is not relieved, medications may be changed, diagnostic tests may be delayed or done as soon as

Nursing Interventions	Rationales
	possible, and surgery may be performed prior to scheduled date or delayed to note resolution of inflammatory changes longer.
Apply pelvic belt traction if prescribed.	Pelvic belt traction is used to help relieve low back pain.
Teach patient how to remove self from pelvic belt.	Patients need to know how to remove the belt/traction if it increases the pain. The patient may be "in 2 h, out 2 h" or similar patterns. Learning how to remove the belt increases the patient's sense of control.
Coordinate planned diagnostic examinations with appropriate personnel or departments.	Coordination lessens delays between departments for optimal care.

▶ NURSING DIAGNOSIS: *Knowledge Deficit*

Related To unfamiliar terms and postoperative self-care or condition

Defining Characteristics

- Unfamiliarity with new terms: automated percutaneous discectomy, laminectomy, herniated nucleus pulposus, ruptured disc, neurovascular checks, laminectomy checks, and others
- Inability to ask questions due to fear or other reason
- Unknown postoperative course and long-term outcome

Patient Outcomes

The patient will

- be able to make decisions about type of surgical procedure after physician's explanations.
- not experience any complications.
- participate actively in self-care.
- understand all newly introduced terms after teaching-learning session.
- undergo removal of herniated nucleus pulposus.

Nursing Interventions	Rationales
Assess patient's understandings after physician's explanations.	Assessment should include use of terms used by physician. Data are used as basis for teaching.
Clarify any unclear or misunderstood explanations.	Patient may need some clarifications related to unfamiliar terms or technique of surgery.
Use pictures, diagrams, or charts as needed.	Patients learn from a variety of visual aids.
Include family members in teaching session.	All involved persons should have similar understandings to lessen anxiety.
Refer to physician, if needed, for additional information.	Several sessions with physician may be needed for full understanding due to unanswered questions.
Teach patient postoperative self-care and expected recovery process.	Being aware of self-care needs helps patient participate actively with recovery process.

▶ NURSING DIAGNOSIS: *High Risk for Altered Peripheral Tissue Perfusion*

Risk Factors
- Pressure on spinal nerves from disc fragments
- Hemorrhage or edema postoperatively
- Surgical trauma from trocar or nucleotome or from laminectomy

Patient Outcomes
The patient will
- have no neurologic or circulatory complications.
- regain pain-free physical mobility after surgery.

Nursing Interventions	Rationales
Assess neurologic/circulatory functions of both lower extremities.	Assessment data provide basis for nursing care.
Compare neurologic/circulatory data with preoperative condition.	Helps determine if surgery was corrective or if benefits are not evident at the time.

Nursing Interventions	Rationales
Continue to do neurovascular or laminectomy checks as prescribed; record and report changes, if negative, to physician.	All nine parts of neurovascular checks should be done to note any untoward signs, such as increase in numbness, pain, or changes in skin color. Neurovascular checks are explained on page 21. Laminectomy checks also include checking muscle/joint strength by pushing and pulling on dorsum and plantar areas of both feet, along with other checks.
Monitor vital signs as prescribed.	A decrease in systolic blood pressure or rise in pulse rates may indicate bleeding at surgical site. An elevated temperature may be indicative of a developing infection, either at the surgical site or elsewhere in the body.
Monitor voiding and measure amounts.	Inability to void or incontinence may indicate injury to nerves controlling bladder functions.
Listen for complaints of headache.	Headache may be related to injury to the dura mater, a developing infection, or decreased spinal fluid levels.
Monitor operative site for evidence of bleeding, hemorrhage, or edema.	Percutaneous discectomy involves insertion of a trocar into the disc space after injection of the local anesthetic, with the patient lying prone on the operating table. A minimal incision of 2 mm permits insertion of the trocar under fluoroscopic control into the disc space. The herniated disc is removed with a nucleotome to aspirate the disc fragments. Edema may develop at the incision site. Bleeding or hemorrhage are uncommon after percutaneous discectomy but may occasionally occur after laminectomy.

▶ NURSING DIAGNOSIS: *Impaired Physical Mobility*

Related To surgical removal of ruptured disc and preoperative pressure on spinal nerves

Defining Characteristics

- Complaints of numbness and weakness of right or left leg and foot
- Radiologic evidence of ruptured disc with multiple fragments
- Hesitant to stand upright with normal lumbar lordosis
- Walks with "straight" back due to muscle spasms and lumbar back pain (lacks lumbar lordosis)

Patient Outcomes

The patient will

- regain usual mobility after recovery from surgery.
- experience relief of back muscle spasms and lumbar pain.

Nursing Interventions	Rationales
Assess ability to turn self in bed with assistance.	Usually can actively help turn from side to side.
Reposition as desired.	Lying on either side is usually more comfortable than lying on back.
Assist to be up in chair as prescribed.	Usually the patient can be up in a chair the day of laminectomy. Discharge to home usually is common 2–4 h after a percutaneous discectomy. Removal of a ruptured disc with a laser also allows same-day discharge.
Encourage the patient to ambulate as able.	Ambulation is usually permitted the day of laminectomy, with assistance if foot or leg numbness persists, or there are lingering effects from anesthesia.
Elevate the head of the bed if desired.	Patients may recline in Fowler's position after open laminectomy or percutaneous discectomy.
Prepare for discharge as prescribed.	Patients are discharged on same day after percutaneous discectomy.

DISCHARGE PLANNING/CONTINUITY OF CARE

- Discuss use of heat or cold applications to relieve muscle spasms if recurring.
- Secure follow-up appointment with physician.
- Provide written guidelines of symptoms to notify physician if they develop, such as fever, drainage, redness, edema, pain, or difficulty breathing.
- Provide written list of do's and don'ts after laminectomy.

REFERENCES

Borenstein, D., & Wiesel, S. (1989). Low back pain: *Medical diagnosis and comprehensive management.* Philadelphia: Saunders.

Deyo, R. A., & Bass, J. E. (1989). Lifestyle and low back pain. The influence of smoking and obesity. *Spine, 14,* 501–506.

Feingold, D. J., Peck, S. A., Reinsma, E. J., & Ruda, S. C. (1991). Complications of lumbar surgery. *Orthopaedic Nursing, 10*(4), 39–58.

Jerva, M. J. (1993). Automated percutaneous lumbar discectomy: A review. *Orthopaedic Nursing, 12*(3), 27–31.

CHEMONUCLEOLYSIS

Chemonucleolysis involves injection of the enzyme chymopapain into the nucleus pulposus, which then, through the processes of breakdown of the protein-carbohydrate complexes and inflammation, will heal with scar tissue in the disc space. Some patients may have sensitivities to this enzyme, which has made its use controversial. The procedure is being done less frequently now than in past years.

▶ NURSING DIAGNOSIS: *High Risk for Injury (Anaphylactic Reaction)*

Risk Factors

- Female gender, positive pregnancy test
- History of allergic reactions to other allergens

Patient Outcomes

The patient will

- experience no allergic reaction to chymopapain.
- undergo chemonucleolysis safely.

Nursing Interventions	Rationales
Assess patient's history for allergic reactions and for possible pregnancy.	Chymopapain breaks down protein-carbohydrate complexes but can cause allergic or anaphylactic reactions in sensitive persons that have resulted in a chemonucleolysis death rate of about 1%.
Clarify, if needed, patient's understanding from physician's explanations of this procedure.	Some patients need repeated explanations for full understanding.

Nursing Interventions	Rationales
Make certain that required blood and serum studies are done, including a complete blood count, bleeding and clotting studies, hematocrit and hemoglobin, electrocardiogram, chest x-ray, and urinalysis.	Each test provides data relevant to patient's health status.
Do usual preoperative preparations of patient according to hospital protocols.	Proper preparations provide a safety measure that the patient is in the best condition to undergo the proposed procedure.
Administer the prescribed preoperative medications, observing the "five rights." Medications commonly given before a chemonucleolysis include diphenhydramine (Benadryl), 50 mg given q4h in three doses the evening prior; methyl prednisolone (Solu-medrol), 250 mg intravenous push 1 h prior to surgery; and cimetidine (Tagamet), 300 mg intravenous over 30 min in the 30 min preceding the surgery.	These medications are given to lessen the possibility of allergic reactions, and the methyl prednisolone also is an anti-inflammatory agent.
Postoperatively, assess patient closely for complaints of shortness of breath, rash, hives or itching, periorbital edema, or voice tightness.	These complaints are signs of allergic or anaphylactic reaction and should be immediately reported to physician.
Monitor vital signs every hour for 8 h, then q2h for next 16 h, then q4h (if still hospitalized).	Decreases in systolic blood pressures, along with increases in pulse and respiratory rates, are untoward signs that may be part of anaphylactic reaction.
Listen for bowel sounds in each abdominal quadrant q4h; ask patient if has passed flatus.	Peristalsis may be slowed from medications or surgery. Bowel sounds should be present and flatus passed prior to oral intake and resumption of diet.
Listen for breath sounds in all lobes of lungs.	Presence of fluid in lungs may be an indication of allergic reaction or of a developing infection.

Nursing Interventions	Rationales
Measure intake and output q8h.	Balances should be nearly alike, taking into consideration insensible losses.
Begin oral intake when bowel sounds are active and patient is expelling flatus.	Oral intake can be tolerated without risk of paralytic ileus if bowel sounds are active, indicating peristalsis is normal.

▶ NURSING DIAGNOSIS: *Impaired Physical Mobility*

Related To postoperative back muscle spasms and back pain

Defining Characteristics

- Complaints of back pain
- Inability to find a position of comfort
- Muscle spasms in area of herniated nucleus pulposus

Patient Outcomes

The patient will

- be relieved of back pain and muscle spasms after medications.
- regain physical mobility by time of discharge to home.

Nursing Interventions	Rationales
Assess severity of back pain (compare with preoperative pain), duration, type, characteristics, and site of pain and muscle spasms.	Postoperatively, the patient may have duller, more localized pain, almost continuously in the back with less or no radiation down legs (if present prior to chemonucleolysis). The pain is related to the injection of the chymopapain into the disc space, which temporarily may increase the pressure in this space. Muscle spasms may or may not be present. They are due to irritation of the chymopapain (Hadjipavlou, Lauder, & Antoniou, 1992).

Nursing Interventions	**Rationales**
Assist the patient to a position of comfort, often side lying, with pillows to back and between legs. The head of the bed may be elevated 30°–45° and the knee gatch may also be elevated 30°–45°.	Side lying with head/knees elevated decreases pressure on back to relieve pain and muscle spasms.
Apply ice or cryotherapy or heating pad to area of injection of chymopapain.	The cold or heat help relieve muscle spasms and pain. The use of heat or cold is optional with the patient who may alternate their use.
Administer prescribed analgesics and muscle-relaxant medications q4h.	These medications provide continuous pain relief and decrease in muscle spasms.
Evaluate effects of ice or heat, analgesics, and muscle relaxants.	These therapies should provide comfort and relief of pain and muscle spasms. If they do not, possibly they may need to be changed or the patient's condition may need to be reported to the physician.
When the patient's condition has stabilized, prepare him or her for discharge: Help patient ambulate to bathroom, assist with donning own clothes, teach patient about oral analgesics and muscle relaxants and their side effects, and secure return appointment for patient to see physician.	The patient must have stable vital signs and no temperature elevation, along with pain and muscle spasms controlled or relieved by medications prior to discharge. The patient should be able to ambulate with assistance and have voided satisfactorily.
Assist patient with self-care as needed.	Patient may need help due to muscle spasms or pain.
Teach patient to report to physician if hives, rash, or edema develop after discharge.	Delayed anaphylactic reaction could, but usually does not, occur after discharge. The patient should be instructed to call for emergency medical care immediately if these symptoms occur at home.

DISCHARGE PLANNING/CONTINUITY OF CARE

- Provide written list of symptoms to report to physician if they occur.
- Secure follow-up visit to physician.
- Provide written instructions for medications, purposes, and expected side effects.

REFERENCES

Chemonucleolysis update (1992). Neurological complications (Bulletin), January 1992. Lincolnshire, IL: Boots Pharmaceuticals.

Chemonucleolysis update (1993). Anaphylaxis (Bulletin), January 1993. Lincolnshire, IL: Boots Pharmaceuticals.

Hadjipavlou, A., Lauder, P., & Antoniou, J. (1992). The effect of chymopapain on low back pain. *Orthopaedic Review, 21*(6), 733–738.

SPINAL FUSION

Spinal fusion, with the use of pedicle screws, bone grafts, or insertion of Harrington, Luque, Cotrel-Dubousset, or other rods, may be done to treat various injuries or deformities. Fusions using rods may be done to treat scoliosis or burst vertebral fractures. Pedicle screws may be used for alignment of vertebrae following flexion distraction or fracture dislocation injuries. Pedicle screws are placed through the transverse processes into the pedicle into the vertebral bodies. Bone grafts may be used along with screws to help fuse vertebral segments after removal of a herniated disc or discs from several intervertebral annular areas. Spinal fusions, when well healed, make the fused areas immobile and solid.

ETIOLOGIES

- Burst, compression, flexion distraction, or fracture dislocation of one or more vertebrae
- Degenerative osteoarthritis or ankylosing spondylitis of vertebral segments
- Herniation of one or more nucleus pulposus
- Spondylolisthesis (slipping forward of vertebral segment)

CLINICAL MANIFESTATIONS

- Congenital defect in back (spondylolisthesis)
- Dull, aching pain in cervical, thoracic, lumbar, or sacral vertebral segments
- Fixed forward flexion of neck or severe kyphosis of thoracic spine
- Herniation of disc with low back pain
- Traumatic injury to vertebra(e) resulting in fracture

CLINICAL/DIAGNOSTIC FINDINGS

- Magnetic resonance imaging (MRI) revealing herniation of one or more intervertebral discs, presence of spondylolisthesis, or scoliosis
- Presence of HLA-B27 antigen diagnostic of ankylosing spondylitis in serum
- Roentgenograms showing marked lipping of vertebral bodies and degeneration of facet joints with osteophytes indicative of osteoarthritis

- Roentgenograms revealing fracture(s) of vertebral bodies, transverse or posterior processes

▶ NURSING DIAGNOSIS: *Impaired Physical Mobility*

Related To spinal fusion using

- bone grafts with spinal screws for ankylosing spondylitis
- pedicular screw fixation of spondylolisthesis
- insertion of Harrington, Luque, Cotrel-Dubousset, or other rods for scoliosis or burst fractures
- pedicle screws for osteoarthritis or fractures of vertebrae

Defining Characteristics

- Operative report stating spinal fusion as listed above under nursing diagnosis
- Pain in lower back with radiation down back of both legs
- Pain in operative sites and incisional areas
- Presence of nasogastric tube
- Presence of thoracic lumbar spine orthosis (TLSO) of molded plastic
- Presence of wound drainage system

Patient Outcomes

The patient will

- apply orthosis properly after teaching.
- maintain stable (intact) spinal fusion when rising or returning to bed by using proper techniques.
- participate in logrolling passively, then actively after period of healing.
- regain mobility with assistance after period of bedrest.

Nursing Interventions	Rationales
Assess operative site and dressing with patient on side.	Data may indicate presence of bleeding or wound drainage system.
Position patient on side using logrolling technique with assistance of another nursing service person.	Initially, and for first 6–7 post-operative days, the patient should be logrolled by two persons with the patient remaining a passive participant until sufficient healing and collagen are present in the operative area for the patient to become more active in repositioning safely. Logrolling prevents twisting of the body and vertebral column, which could cause disruption of the

Nursing Interventions	Rationales
	surgical repair. During passive logrolling, the patient holds self stiff while being turned to the side by one nurse pulling with a hand on the far shoulder and hip. The second nurse pushes the patient at the same time to help turn, then carefully pulls lowermost shoulder and hip areas to align body. Pillows are placed to the back and between the legs to help maintain the side-lying position.
Massage back, shoulders, and hips when on side.	Massage eases muscle strain and pain due to length of surgical repair and recovery period. Massage also brings circulation to area to aid healing and to maintain healthy skin areas.
Apply TSLO orthosis or other brace, if prescribed.	An orthosis or brace helps the patient maintain a stable vertebral column to aid healing and prevent loss of reduction or repair.
When allowed up, assist patient to sit at bedside with orthosis or brace on, then assist to be up in a chair.	Assistance is required so patient does not overstrain operative internal fixation devices, which could cause loss of operative repair or placement.
Assist patient to ambulate with orthosis or brace.	Ambulation helps patient regain strength and is a positive step toward recovery.
Encourage patient to do active dorsiflexion/plantarflexion and circumduction exercises of feet and ankles q2h.	Active ankle and foot exercises increase circulation and venous return and prevent venous stasis.
Teach patient to use proper body mechanics for lifting.	Use of proper body mechanics prevents new injuries to back when healing and later.
Teach patient use of ambulatory aids, if prescribed.	An ambulatory aid lends security and safety to patient's ambulation until it can be done independently.

▶ NURSING DIAGNOSIS: *Altered Peripheral Tissue Perfusion*

Related To immobility and surgical trauma

Defining Characteristics

- Bedrest for 1–3 days or longer
- Lengthy surgical procedure for spinal instrumentation or fusion
- Removal of cancellous bone tissues for use as bone grafts to spine from iliac crest or tibia

Patient Outcomes

The patient will

- experience no deep-vein thrombosis.
- regain satisfactory peripheral tissue perfusion after healing.
- regain normal ranges of neurovascular functions.
- regain satisfactory ambulation and mobility.

Nursing Interventions	Rationales
Assess neurovascular functions through "laminectomy checks": Assess legs and feet for peripheral pulses, capillary refill, color, temperature, edema, pain, numbness or tingling, and motor strength or muscle strength, and compare findings in both extremities. Push-pull strength may also be done to check muscle strength.	Results of these checks provide data related to adequacy of peripheral tissue perfusion and oxygenation. There will usually be some edema of one or both extremities, some motor/muscle weakness, some slight to moderate numbness or tingling, and moderate to severe pain in the iliac crest or tibia in bone graft donor site. The motor and sensory changes should return to normal in 24–48 h. Assessments should be done hourly initially for 8 h, then q2–3h, and finally q4h. Capillary refill should be 2–4 s. All peripheral pulses should be present.
Encourage patient to do ankle/foot dorsiflexion/plantarflexion and circumduction exercises q2h.	These exercises increase venous return to decrease venous stasis and edema formation.
Perform Homan test by dorsiflexing each foot toward calf.	This technique is one check for thrombophlebitis.
Logroll patient from side to side q2h.	Changing positions aids general circulation and oxygenation by relieving pressure and decreasing

Nursing Interventions	Rationales
	muscle tension. Use pillows to help patient maintain proper positions.
Administer narcotic analgesics or monitor use of patient-controlled analgesia (PCA) pump q3–4h around the clock initially, and administer prescribed muscle-relaxant medications.	The patient may complain of moderate to severe pain in donor bone graft site due to bleeding/pressure in this site, with less pain in operative site.
Assist patient to apply orthosis or back brace when allowed up. Increase ambulation as condition permits.	Bedrest varies with patient's condition and operative procedure. Ambulation facilitates peripheral circulation, decreases edema, and provides positive input to aid recovery.
Apply elastic or antithrombotic hose, if prescribed.	Use of such hose constricts superficial vessels to prevent venous stasis.

▶ NURSING DIAGNOSIS: *Impaired skin integrity*

Related To long incisional area, drain in wound, presence of sutures or skin clips, and donor bone graft site

Defining Characteristics

- Incisional areas (operative site and donor site) closed with skin clips or sutures
- Wound drain at lower end of incision

Patient Outcomes

The patient will

- experience wound healing without dehiscence (wound opening up) or infection.
- have satisfactory wound drainage without stasis.
- not develop pressure areas or skin excoriation from orthosis or brace.
- tolerate pressure and pain from donor site.

Nursing Interventions	Rationales
Assess all skin areas, incision, and donor sites for redness, edema,	Signs of pressure include redness or white areas over bony prominences.

Nursing Interventions	**Rationales**
numbness, excoriation, or open areas.	Initially, incisional/donor sites may be red, edematous, and painful due to inflammation to aid healing. Drainage may initially be sanguineous, then become serosanguineous, and finally become clear. The amount of drainage varies from 100 to 200 mL totally until drain is removed. If suction in wound, recompress suction after emptying drainage chamber.
Using aseptic technique, change wound/donor dressings as prescribed by physician.	Presence of drainage on dressings may foster bacterial growth leading to infection. Clean drainage from wounds and reapply dressings as needed.
Reposition patient q2h.	Repositioning increases circulation to all skin areas to prevent skin breakdown or pressure areas.
Help patient put on T-shirt before applying orthosis or brace.	Use of a T-shirt prevents rubbing of brace or orthosis directly on skin plus absorbs perspiration to lessen skin maceration.
Massage skin areas several times daily.	Massage increases circulation to decrease formation of pressure areas.
Assist with removal of or remove skin clips or sutures, if nursing responsibility.	Nurses may remove skin clips or sutures in some hospitals or clinics, whereas in some areas removal is a physician's responsibility.
Observe wound areas for signs of opening or dehiscence.	Dehiscence may be related to too early removal of skin clips or sutures, poor nutrition, or decreased collagen formation in the patient. Small areas of dehiscence, may be closed with steristrips or butterfly dressings, but if a large area has dehisced, the wound may need to be resutured and retention sutures may have to be added until the wound has healed well.

Nursing Interventions	Rationales
Observe wound sites and drainage for signs of infection such as purulent drainage, marked redness, edema, increase in pain, abscess formation, or dehiscence.	Wound infection is a severe complication after insertion of spinal rods or bone grafts, as the infection can spread to the coverings of the spinal cord. At times, the metallic rods or bone grafts may need to be removed to aid clearing of the infection.

▶ NURSING DIAGNOSIS: *Impaired Gas Exchange*

Related To bedrest, anesthesia, and immobility

Defining Characteristics

- Lengthy anesthesia period
- Preoperative bedrest due to fracture of vertebrae, skeletal traction, or concomitant injuries
- Postoperative bedrest in flat position in bed
- Scoliosis with curvature beyond 40°

Patient Outcomes

The patient will

- develop no pulmonary complications.
- perform deep-breathing exercises and reach goals for incentive spirometer.
- regain full lung expansion and normal gas exchange.

Nursing Interventions	Rationales
Assess respiratory rates and depth and presence of dyspnea, cough, and breath sounds.	Increased respiratory rates, splinting or shallow breathing, dyspnea or shortness of breath plus a productive cough with yellow or green sputum, and decreased breath sounds are all signs of pulmonary infection, pneumonia, or atelectasis.
Encourage deep-breathing exercises q2h plus use of incentive spirometer with increasing depth goals.	Deep breathing helps perfuse lung alveoli with oxygen and removal of carbon dioxide. Some areas of the

Nursing Interventions	Rationales
	lung may have been compromised preoperatively due to scoliosis curve or fractured vertebra and postoperatively can be more fully perfused with deep breathing or use of incentive spirometer to increase depth of inhalations.
Monitor body temperature q4h.	Infection in lungs is reflected by temperature elevations and decreased or absent breath sounds.
When permitted, assist patient to be up and ambulate with use of orthosis or brace.	Ambulation increases deep breathing and perfusion of all body cells.
Monitor patient for mental alertness and skin color changes (dusky or bluish color).	Decreased or change in consciousness plus dusky or cyanotic skin changes are signs of decreased oxygenation.

▶ NURSING DIAGNOSIS: *Acute Pain*

Related To surgical trauma, incision, donor site, and muscle stretching

Defining Characteristics

- Frequently asks for pain medication or uses PCA to "lock-out" stage
- Marked bruising at donor site for bone graft
- Long incision over vertebral column
- Straightening of scoliosis curve with muscle stretching on previous curve side

Patient Outcomes

The patient will

- have pain relieved with prescribed medications.
- have muscle lengthening without muscle spasms.
- have soreness and bruising of donor site relieved as inflammation resolves.

Nursing Interventions	Rationales
Assess for presence, type, sites, severity, and duration of pain.	The amount and severity of pain may vary among individuals, but

Nursing Interventions	Rationales
	the majority of persons after spinal fusion or instrumentation complain of fairly severe, almost constant pain and require around-the-clock medications for pain to be controlled. Muscle-relaxant medications may be given between narcotic dosages to aid pain relief. As inflammation decreases and healing proceeds, the patient becomes more pain free and able to control pain with milder narcotic analgesics, including oxycodone, or with nonnarcotic analgesics, such as acetaminophen or ibuprofen.
Listen to patient's complaints of pain, its duration and type, and its decrease over time.	At times, if patient's pain is not controlled, the strength and/or kind of narcotic analgesic may need to be changed. Listening to the patient's complaints reassures the patient that concerns will be dealt with. Painful periods should decrease as inflammatory changes abate and healing progresses. Pain that persists over an uncommonly long period may be indicative of disruption of operative repair or other complication.
Reposition patient q2h.	Repositioning relieves tired, aching, sore or painful muscles, joints, and other tissues by relieving pressure on nerve endings.
Monitor effects of medication to achieve relief of pain.	Narcotics decrease perception of pain and should provide satisfactory pain relief if given around the clock to help maintain therapeutic blood levels of medication. The addition of muscle relaxant and anti-inflammatory medications may enhance pain relief.

Nursing Interventions	Rationales
Monitor complaints of pain in "unusual" sites such as muscles of thigh or leg.	These complaints may be related to development of compartment syndrome or thrombophlebitis.
Monitor wound healing over time.	Pain in wound area should decrease as healing proceeds. An increase in pain in wound area may be related to an infection, such as an abscess, or from pressure on nerve endings.

▶ NURSING DIAGNOSIS: *High Risk for Injury*

Risk Factors

- Misplacement of screws or rods without adequate purchase (attachment) at time of surgery
- Poor nutritional status with anemia
- Twisting of spinal column when turning or when not wearing brace or orthosis

Patient Outcomes

The patient will

- experience no disruption of fixation devices or grafts.
- learn proper application of orthosis or brace.
- understand reasons for and methods of logrolling.

Nursing Interventions	Rationales
Assess body alignment and position and security of brace or orthosis.	Body alignment should be as near normal as possible. The orthosis or brace should fit fairly snugly and be secured closed when in use. It should not permit the patient to twist vertebral column.
Monitor placement of bed frame in down or flat position and use of pillows.	Following a spinal fusion the patient is kept flat for varying periods postoperatively to help maintain the operative repair, especially if screws are not used to hold grafted bones.

Nursing Interventions	Rationales
Logroll patient with assistance until patient can participate more actively in turning.	Logrolling helps maintain the vertebral column in a straight, untwisted line. In about 72 h postoperatively, the patient may be able to take a more active role in the logrolling process.
Listen to patient's statements of hearing or feeling something "pop," having a bulge in back, not being able to move legs or arms, or other complaints.	These statements may be related to loss of operative correction or wound hematoma or abscess or other concern.
Provide needed equipment such as straight-backed chair, cane or crutches, and long-handled reachers, as needed.	Use of proper ambulatory aids plus assistive devices helps prevent injury or disruption of operative repair.
Teach patient how to apply orthosis or brace and how to use ambulatory aid or assistive devices.	Being able to use equipment safely and properly increases patient's self-confidence, provides safety in care, and aids compliance.

▶ NURSING DIAGNOSIS: *Constipation*

Related To anesthesia, bedrest, or immobility

Defining Characteristics

- Abdominal fullness and distention
- Decreased bowel sounds
- Inability to have normal bowel movement
- Narcotic usage q4h

Patient Outcomes

The patient will

- be able to have nonconstipated bowel movement.
- be relieved of abdominal distention and fullness.
- regain normal bowel sounds.

Nursing Interventions	Rationales
Assess for bowel sounds, abdominal distention, and last bowel movement.	Bowel sounds should be low pitched and rumbling and be heard in all four quadrants of abdomen. Sounds are related to peristalsis and are usually heard every 30 s.
Measure abdominal girth; percuss for sounds related to ileus.	Abdominal girth will increase with abdominal distention and ileus. Sounds on percussion will be hollow if ileus is present. Narcotics constrict sphincters, making defecation difficult.
Irrigate nasogastric tube, if present, q4h.	Irrigation helps maintain patency of tube.
If no bowel movement for several days postoperatively, insert rectal suppository, if prescribed, prior to attempting to have bowel movement.	Suppositories help moisten and soften fecal mass to aid passage.
Begin food and fluid intake slowly, when prescribed.	Beginning slowly helps gastrointestinal tract regain functions and prevents gastric distention or vomiting.
Administer stool softener or laxative orally at bedtime, if prescribed.	Use of a stool softener and laxative aids evacuation of fecal mass.
Encourage intake of high-fiber foods and fluid intake to 3,000 mL daily.	High-fiber foods provide bulk to increase fecal mass, and fluids provide lubrication to aid defecation.
Examine amount, color, and consistency of stool.	Stool should be brown, soft formed, and of a moderate amount, partially related to intake.

▶ NURSING DIAGNOSIS: *Altered Urinary Output*

Related To surgical trauma, bedrest, anesthesia, and immobility

Defining Characteristics

- Has enlarged prostate or cystocele
- Inability to void from flat-bed position
- Intake only of intravenous fluids

Patient Outcomes

The patient will

- be able to void in bedside commode.
- not develop urinary tract infection.
- not need to be catheterized more than once.

Nursing Interventions	Rationales
Assess bladder for feeling of fullness or distention.	A full bladder will be distended and patient may have urgency to void.
If permitted to be up, apply brace or orthosis and assist patient to bedside commode.	The upright position aids gravity to permit emptying of bladder.
If on bedrest, place "fracture" bed pan under patient or place urinal; facilitate voiding by running water in sink, having patient put fingers in warm water, or pouring warm water over perineum (female patient only).	Use of these techniques relaxes bladder sphincters to aid voiding.
If patient unable to void in 10–12 h postoperatively, secure prescription for medication such as bethanechol (Urecholine) to aid voiding or catheterize patient.	Bethanechol relaxes bladder sphincter to aid voiding. Catheterization may be needed to prevent overdistention of bladder.
Monitor fluid intake and output.	Fluid intake of 3,000 mL over 24 h aids renal perfusion and formation of urine.

▶ NURSING DIAGNOSIS: *Chronic Pain*

Related To inadequate knowledge of pain management, inflammatory process, or joint degeneration

Defining Characteristics

- Complains of persistent pain in low back 6 months after percutaneous discectomy
- Works part time only, not full time
- Walks with hands applying pressure on lower back area
- Nonunion of fractured bone

Patient Outcomes

The patient will

- become an active participant in pain control measures.
- verbalize wish to experience relief of pain.
- use a variety of measures to control pain.
- identify activities that increase or decrease pain.

Nursing Interventions	Rationales
Assess patient's pain experiences, expressions of pain, and previous measures used to control pain.	Pain experiences and expressions vary among individuals, and control measures also vary. Expressions of pain may include crying, anger, sadness, harsh words against health team members, or other expressions.
Assess patient's demeanor and positions while describing pain experiences.	Patient may moan, wince, frown, slump in chair, hold lumbar area of back, pace, or ask to lie down.
Use caution to maintain patient's trust.	Pain is "what the patient says it is," according to McCaffery & Beebe (1989). Some patients in chronic pain may be distrustful or suspicious that health care personnel may not believe them based on past experiences.
Discuss methods to record patient's pain experiences.	Patients may use a visual display of 0–10 or 0–5 on a vertical or horizontal line. They may also record dates, times, and effect of measures to relieve the pain in a written log or diary. These measures increase the patient's sense of control.
Discuss effects of medications used to relieve patient's pain.	Medications used for chronic pain include nonnarcotic analgesics and nonsteroidal anti-inflammatory drugs.
Discuss techniques to relieve pain, such as visualization, relaxation, biofeedback, use of heat or cold, and rest.	These techniques may be used intermittently, simultaneously, or consecutively, according to patient's willingness to use them.

Nursing Interventions	Rationales
	Each must be used more than once for its effects to be noted or benefits received.
Teach how to do pain control techniques.	Education is needed for unfamiliar techniques for best results, safety, and patient comfort.
Discuss patient's perceptions of referral to pain clinic and "back school."	Personnel in pain clinics and "back school" help patients deal with chronic pain experiences using specific exercises and other techniques found to be beneficial by patients.
Identify and record activities that cause, increase, or decrease pain.	Understanding what activities alter pain experiences is beneficial to patient and health team members.
Assist patient to identify effective mechanisms for coping with chronic pain.	
Administer prescribed analgesics/anti-inflammatory medications.	Nonnarcotic and anti-inflammatory medications help provide relief for chronic pain episodes.

DISCHARGE PLANNING/CONTINUITY OF CARE

- Refer to home care nurses for wound care, ambulation, activities for daily living, and sexual activity as needed.
- Refer to dietitian for dietary management related to weight control or presence of brace or orthosis.
- Provide written instructions for medication regimen, purposes, and side effects; review as needed.
- Provide follow-up appointment with physician.

REFERENCES

Bridwell, K. H. (1988). Cotrel-Dubousset instrumentation. *Orthopaedic Nursing, 7*(1), 11–16.

Brosnan, H., & Berda, P. Pedicle screw fixation in the lumbar spine. *Orthopaedic Nursing, 9*(6), 22–32.

Ficner, H. B. (1993). Revision surgery in adult scoliosis patient. *Orthopaedic Nursing, 12*(2), 23–32.

McCaffery, M., & Beebe, A. (1989). *Pain: Clinical manual for nursing practice.* St. Louis: C.V. Mosby.

Richardson, A. B., Taylor, M. L., & Murphree, Beth. (1990). TSRH instrumentation: Evolution of a new system. *Orthopaedic Nursing, 9*(6), 15–21.

Song, K. & Herring, J. A. (1993). Early recognition and assessment of idiopathic scoliosis. *Journal of Musculoskeletal Medicine, 10*(4), 63–80.

Tepper, G. (1992). Spinal fusion today. *Orthopedic Special Edition, 1*(8), 1, 4.

Complications in Orthopaedics

Complications are undesirable happenings in any illness, but in orthopaedics, complications are especially unwanted because of the many tissues that could be involved. Complications can affect the skin in or around a soft tissue injury, subcutaneous muscles, ligaments, tendons around a joint, and the joint or enclosed bone or bones. Complications may be fairly easy to cure, such as cellulitis, or very difficult, such as infections of a joint or a bone involving osteomyelitis. Prostheses used for retention of fracture reductions can become infected or loosened, as can prostheses used for total joint repairs. Infections and loosening are common complications with orthopaedic patients, as are other complications, such as pulmonary or fat embolism and compartment syndrome, which may be followed by Volkmann ischemic contracture.

INFECTION FOLLOWING TOTAL JOINT ARTHROPLASTY

Infection is always a possibility whenever the skin and joint tissues are opened for a surgical corrective procedure, such as a total joint arthroplasty. With over 250,000 total hip arthroplasties and 175,000 total knee arthroplasties done yearly (Goldberg, 1992), it is highly likely that there will be infections in either of these joints, as well as in lesser repaired joints such as the shoulder, ankle, elbow, or wrist. A postoperative infection is a devastating complication: highly morbid at best, potentially fatal at worst (Kelman, Roland, & Beagley, 1993). The infection can occur in the immediate postoperative period or in the months (up to 1 year) after arthroplasty.

ETIOLOGIES

- Gram negative organisms such as *Pseudomonas aeruginosa, Escherichia coli, Klebsiella,* and *Proteus vulgaris*
- Gram positive organisms such as *Staphylococcus aureus* or *S. epidermidis, Streptococcus,* of beta-hemolytic species
- Presence of rheumatoid arthritis with previous hip surgery

CLINICAL MANIFESTATIONS

- Drainage from wound
- Fever
- Limp
- Pain in affected hip

CLINICAL/DIAGNOSTIC FINDINGS

- Elevated white blood cell (WBC) count (>7,000/mm^3)
- Elevated sedimentation rate
- Physical examination of red, tender, draining hip revealing small fistulous track with purulent drainage
- Spiking temperature > 101 F (38.3 C)

▶ NURSING DIAGNOSIS: *High Risk for Infection*

Risk Factors

- Corticosteroid and methotrexate treatment for rheumatoid arthritis
- Draining fistulous track in operative joint
- Indwelling Foley catheter
- Older adult with decreased immune response
- Status post–total joint replacement

Patient Outcomes

The patient will

- become infection free following treatments.
- not develop resistance to antibiotics used for treatment.
- not require removal of prostheses.

Nursing Interventions	Rationales
Assess condition of patient: age, postoperative time frame, hip drainage, temperature, and vital signs.	Older persons with chronic illness, such as rheumatoid arthritis and diabetes, have decreased resistance to infection. Deep-wound infection often occurs in the immediate postoperative period in up to 1% or more of total hip arthroplasties (Harris & Barrack, 1993). An elevated body temperature is one indicator of infection. If septicemia is present, the other vital signs may fluctuate, with gram positive or gram negative septicemia strong probabilities.
Using universal precautions and aseptic technique, secure a culture specimen of the wound drainage.	A wound culture should be done to determine, if possible, the nature of the infection and causative organism(s).
Consult with dietitian for nutritional assessment of patient.	Persons with rheumatoid arthritis, having been treated with corticosteroids and methotrexate, may be malnourished and anemic, making them more prone to infection.
Monitor laboratory data related to total protein levels, albumin and	Malnourished persons have decreased total protein, albumin,

Nursing Interventions	Rationales
globulin levels, hemoglobin, and WBC and differential cell counts.	and globulin levels, making them more prone to infections. If their hemoglobin is low, they cannot carry as much oxygen, and if the WBC and certain differential cell counts are lower (lymphocytes, monocytes, and neutrophils), they cannot fight infections as well.
Monitor intake and output.	If Foley catheter had been in bladder postoperatively, it may have been the source of infection (Ritter, Faris, & Keating, 1989). Intake and output (I&O) provide vital hydration and fluid balance information.
Monitor amount, type, color, and odor of drainage and condition of wound (fistulous track enlarging?).	If drainage is increasing, the infection may be worsening and may necessitate removal of prostheses, especially if infection is from virulent gram negative (e.g., Pseudomonas) organisms (Kelman et al., 1993).
Monitor results of erythrocyte sedimentation rates.	Test values should return to normal (Cushner, 1992); approximately 6 months postoperatively. A rate that remains 40 mm/h is highly suggestive of infection (Harris & Barrack, 1993).
Monitor results of roentgen examinations of operative joint.	Rapid development of continuous radiolucency > 2 mm within the first year is a strong indicator of infection (Harris & Barrack, 1993). Also, focal lysis (destruction), extensive nonfocal lysis, endosteal scalloping, and/or periostitis are other signs of infection (Harris & Barrack, 1993).
Administer prescribed antibiotics q6–8h.	Antibiotics initially may be given intravenously q6–8h to establish a therapeutic blood level. After several days or weeks, the route may be switched to oral administration

Nursing Interventions	Rationales
	for up to 1 year or longer, if tolerated. The specific antibiotic varies according to culture and sensitivity data.
Weigh patient daily, especially if parenteral nutrition and medication have been instituted.	Infection with spiking fevers is a very debilitating condition and patients may lose weight from decreased intake and appetite. Patients may be started on parenteral nutrition to help gain weight.
Observe patient's color or color changes, if they occur.	The skin becomes markedly reddened in gram positive septicemia and gray-ashen in gram negative septicemia. These changes are related to the effects of exotoxins and endotoxins on the capillaries.
Assist with aspiration of infected joint.	Aspiration of the joint is an important diagnostic determination of joint sepsis.

▶ NURSING DIAGNOSIS: *Acute Pain*

Related To pressure of mass purulent drainage

Defining Characteristics

- Pain with sudden onset
- Pain occurring during rest or at night
- Pain relieved after administration of antibiotics
- Pain on weight bearing

Patient Outcomes

The patient will

- be relieved of postoperative (or later) pain occurrences.
- be able to sleep all night without experiencing pain.
- experience no pain on weight bearing after treatments.

Nursing Interventions	Rationales
Assess type, amount, time of, and duration of pain occurrences.	Data are needed to determine source of pain and possible causes. Pain that occurs at night or at rest is thought to be related to infection (Harris and Barrack, 1993).
Monitor effects of position changes on pain experiences.	Changing positions relaxes sore or crampy muscles and relieves some pain.
Administer analgesics as prescribed.	Analgesics lessen perception of pain and painful episodes.
Monitor results of roentgen studies of operative joint.	Roentgen studies may show loosening secondary to presence of infection. Persistent pain after a cemented total hip replacement has been found to be an indicator of chronic indolent infection in many cases (Harris and Barrack, 1993).
Observe all orifices for drainage which may cause pain and inflammation.	Inflammatory signs are changes in color, edema, and increased temperature and pain. Increased drainage is a sign of inflammation in one or more orifices.
Encourage patient to use an ambulatory aid, such as a walker, cane, or crutches.	Use of an ambulatory aid relieves pressure of weight bearing on painful tissues.

▶ NURSING DIAGNOSIS: *Impaired Physical Mobility*

Related To pain and joint infection

Defining Characteristics

- Presence of limp on weight bearing
- Unable to walk any distance without pain or limp

Patient Outcomes

The patient will

- ambulate without a limp.
- regain painless ambulation.

Nursing Interventions	Rationales
Assess mobility, when limp occurs, and relationship of pain with ambulation.	Assessment data provide basis for further treatments and nursing care.
Encourage exercises to hip and leg.	Full recovery after a total hip replacement requires that specific exercises be performed for 3–6 months postoperatively to regain muscle strength.
Encourage ambulation to the point of pain or encourage use of ambulatory aid.	At times, ambulating to the point of pain is a positive move for the patient and helps regain confidence.
Observe effects of administration of antibiotics to relieve infection, elevated temperature, and drainage.	If infection is controlled or overcome with proper antibiotics, the patient should be able to walk more easily if prostheses are intact in hip joint.
Observe patient's use of ambulatory aids for proper technique.	The patient may not use proper technique even though properly taught previously.
Seek consultation with physical therapists.	Specialists have current information for patient's benefit.
Discuss side effects of antibiotics and analgesics.	Side effects of both types of medications include headache, nausea, vomiting, diarrhea or constipation, and at times, depending on the medication, dizziness, which can affect ambulation.

▶ NURSING DIAGNOSIS: *High Risk for Additional Injury*

Risk Factors

- Cemented or uncemented prosthetic parts
- Presence of infection
- Roentgen evidence of osteolysis

Patient Outcomes

The patient will

- have minimal osteolysis.
- not have loosening that requires reoperation.

Nursing Interventions	**Rationales**
Assess ambulation and limp.	Patient may limp related to loosening or subsidence of prosthesis in femur (subsidence is settling of prosthesis farther down shaft of femur from loss of bone stock, which can lead to joint instability.
Observe findings of roentgen studies.	Development of a continuous radiolucent zone of ≥ 2 mm has been found to be a reliable indicator of loosening (Harris and Barrack, 1993). Additionally a distinct line at the prosthesis-cement interface is a virtual guarantee of component loosening (Harris and Barrack, 1993). The line represents debonding of the stem of the femoral prosthesis from the cement mantle. If an uncemented prosthesis was used, subsidence is the single most important indicator of loosening or instability (Harris and Barrack, 1993). Osteolysis is loss of bone stock that can occur in cemented or uncemented prostheses, at times requiring removal and insertion of a new prosthesis. Osteolysis has also been associated with development of aggressive granulomas involving both the acetabular and femoral components (Harris and Barrack, 1993). Osteolysis also occurs from polyethylene wear debris contributing to loosening of the prostheses and failure of the fixation (Huo, Salvati, & Buly, 1991).
Discuss possibility of further diagnostic tests, such as an arthrogram.	An arthrogram involves injection of a radiopaque solution which outlines the joint and prostheses to help determine presence of loosening, although this examination may have false positives or false negatives. However, if the contrast

Nursing Interventions	Rationales
	medium penetrates the bone-cement interface as far as the superior medial aspect of the acetabular cup, it is highly probable the acetabular component is loosened. On the femoral side, if the contrast medium penetrates the bone-cement interface 1–2 cm, the component is loosened (Harris and Barrack, 1993). Friction between the mated metal and polyethylene surfaces is a major cause of polyethylene wear and particle deposition, which can also lead to development of granulomas and loosening (Cuckler, 1990).
	Once loosened, the prostheses are usually removed through a revision total joint arthroplasty as previously discussed.

DISCHARGE PLANNING/CONTINUITY OF CARE

- Make appointment for return to physician.
- Refer to home care nurses for follow-up wound care and ambulation.

REFERENCES

Comadoll, J. L., Gustilio, R. B., & Rockwold, G. L. (1991). Symptomatic intracranial meningiomas after total joint replacement. *Orthopedics, 14*(3), 347–351.

Cuckler, J. M. (1990). Articular wear in total joint arthroplasty: Biologic effects and clinical consequences. *University of Pennsylvania Orthopaedic Journal, 6*(spring), 12–15.

Cushner, F. D., & Morwessel, R. M. (1992). Myositis ossificans traumatica. *Orthopaedic Review, 21*(11), 1319–1326.

Engh, C. A. (1991). Focus on the hip. *Orthopedic and Sports Medicine News, 2*(6), 1, 7.

Goldberg, V. M. (1992). Excellent TKR results noted after neutral alignment. *Orthopedic Special Edition, 1*(9), 12–13.

Harris, W. H., & Barrack, R. L. (1993). Developments in diagnosis of the painful total hip replacement. *Orthopaedic Review, 22*(4), 439–447.

Huo, M. H., Salvati, E. A., & Buly, R. L. (1991). Wear debris in cemented total hip arthroplasty. *Orthopedics, 14*(3), 335–340.

Kelman, G. J., Roland, G. C., & Beagley, M. J. (1993). Acute *Pseudomonas* infection following total hip replacement. *Orthopedics, 16*(2), 209–212.

Ritter, M. A., Faris, P. M., & Keating, E. M. (1989). Urinary tract catheterization protocols following total joint arthroplasty. *Orthopedics, 12*(8), 1085–1087.

COMPARTMENT SYNDROME

Compartment syndrome is an elevation in the venous pressures within a muscle compartment. A compartment consists of muscles and at least one artery, vein, and nerve, all enclosed in fascia, muscle, or bone. Venous pressures rise in the presence of bleeding into a muscle that can occur after a fracture. The rising pressures compromise arterial inflow and the viability and functions of the affected tissues. Thirty-eight compartments are found in the extremities, which are more prone to developing acute compartment syndrome than those in the trunk (Ross, 1991). The compartments in the lower leg and those in the forearm are two common sites for this syndrome. The average time between initial trauma and development of symptoms is 2 h (Ross, 1991).

ETIOLOGIES

- Edema or bleeding into a compartment
- External pressure from a tight cast or dressings
- Presence of pressurized antishock garments
- Persistent exercising

CLINICAL MANIFESTATIONS

- Increase in interstitial fluids causing edema
- Edema increasing intracompartmental pressure
- Arterial spasm from decreased arterial inflow and compression of arterioles
- Tissue ischemia from decreased arterial inflow

CLINICAL/DIAGNOSTIC FINDINGS

- History of soft tissue/bone trauma to an extremity
- Physical examination showing marked edema of injured limb
- Arterial blood pressure readings lower than normal
- Elevated interstitial pressures
- Increased pain on passive movement of digits/toes

▶ NURSING DIAGNOSIS: *High Risk for Additional Injury*

Risk Factors

- Blood vessel damage secondary to above conditions
- Crush injury to extremity
- One or more fractured bones
- Long leg or forearm cast including elbow

Patient Outcomes

The patient will

- have no irreversible muscle/skin/vessel damage secondary to elevated compartment pressures.
- have venous compartment pressures return to normal levels.
- undergo successful fasciotomy or have cast bivalved.

Nursing Interventions	Rationales
Assess extremity for edema, color of tissues, and capillary refill.	Presence of edema, slow (4–6 s) capillary refill, and pallor in tissues are all signs of venous or arterial compromise.
Measure compartment pressures (if no obstruction of cast).	Normal compartment pressures are 10–20 mm venous pressure. Pressures > 25–30 mm are considered elevated.
Notify physician if venous pressure is steadily rising on successive readings.	Once venous pressures approach 30 mm, there will be irreversible ischemic changes in 4–6 h unless the pressure is relieved.
Secure permission to bivalve cast, if present, and if within nursing's role in institution.	Bivalving the cast releases the constricting cast and can permit venous pressures to decrease.
Elevate extremity on pillow.	Elevation increases venous return, thereby lessening edema and pressures.

▶ NURSING DIAGNOSIS: *Acute Pain*

Related To developing compartment syndrome

Patient Outcomes

The patient will

- be relieved of acute pain with treatments and analgesics.
- be able to describe severity of pain.

Nursing Interventions	Rationales
Assess type, duration, sites, and characteristics of patient's pain.	Data from assessments provide information for care.
Perform passive extension of fingers or toes.	Patient complaint of a marked increase in pain, beyond that expected, is one major sign of compartment syndrome.
Observe for weakness or paralysis of digits or toes.	Weakness or paralysis may indicate increased venous pressure on muscle functions.
Observe sensory functions of involved tissues.	Changes in ability to sense pin pricks or loss of sensation are signs of increased pressure.
Observe medication requirements and total amount of narcotic analgesics administered.	More frequent need and larger doses beyond "normal" are signs of pressure on muscles and ischemia. Pain is a sign of anoxia, which is a sign of decreased arterial inflow.
Monitor compartment pressures every hour and notify physician if pressures are rising.	Every hour readings are required, as pressures may increase unsafely if readings are delayed for a longer time.
Administer narcotic analgesic as prescribed.	Narcotic analgesics lessen pain sufficiently to permit the patient to tolerate the remaining pain; however, pain greater than that expected or requiring more medication than usual or normal is a sign of compartment syndrome.
Prepare the patient for fasciotomy if scheduled.	Fasciotomy is opening of the fascia covering the affected muscle. More than one fascial covering may be opened. Fasciotomy allows the muscle to swell and lowers pressures.

▶ NURSING DIAGNOSIS: *High Risk for Infection*

Risk Factors

- Concomitant fracture necessitating immune responses prior to fasciotomy
- Frequent dressing changes required
- Open wound

Patient Outcomes

The patient will

- experience only slight increases in white blood cell (WBC) counts.
- have no elevations of temperatures > 99 F (37.2 C).
- have only serosanguineous to serous drainage from sites.
- not develop an infection in fasciotomy site(s).

Nursing Interventions	Rationales
Assess wound sites for signs of infection: marked tenderness, increase in local tissue warmth, edema, and purulent drainage.	These are all signs of infection.
Monitor vital signs and temperature q2–4h.	Increases in pulse rates, respiration, and temperatures are related to the body's defense against pathogens.
Using universal precautions and aseptic technique, change dressings over fasciotomy sites or over skin grafts if used to close wound.	Precautions are required to prevent introducing pathogens to a patient with lowered resistance. Skin grafts may be placed to cover the enlarged muscle mass as the fascia could be too tight if closed over the muscle mass.
Teach patient signs of infection to report to physician.	Signs or symptoms reported include fever, chills, increased pain, tenderness or warmth at wound site, and presence of drainage.

▶ NURSING DIAGNOSIS: *Knowledge Deficit*

Related To unfamiliar terms, treatments, and outcomes

Defining Characteristics

- Frequent checks of peripheral motor/sensory functions
- Multiple diagnostic examinations

- Sudden trauma with injury to muscles, bone, and skin
- Uncertain outcome
- Unfamiliar terms: compartment syndrome, venous pressures, fasciotomy, bivalving of cast

Patient Outcomes

The patient will

- develop knowledge and understanding of injury and terms.
- participate as actively as condition permits in diagnostic and treatment plan.
- understand purposes of treatments to lower venous pressures.

Nursing Interventions	Rationales
Assess patient's understanding of terms, such as fractured tibia (or radius and ulna) and crush injury and venous pressures used during physician's visit.	Data help determine if additional clarification or teaching is needed.
Use charts, pictures, or other visual aids as needed if clarification is required.	Learning is individualized and is facilitated with visual aids.
Describe nursing care prior to doing it, as when preparing to do neurovascular checks or when preparing patient for roentgenograms or other diagnostic examinations.	Patients can accept and participate more easily if they know the reasons and steps of upcoming care.
Discuss reasons for frequent neurovascular checks and readings of compartment monitoring.	Prior knowledge of events lessens anxiety and helps patient cooperate.
Teach patient symptoms that should be reported to nursing staff.	Prompt reporting helps assure minimal delay in care to relieve untoward symptoms.
Clarify postfasciotomy care, if done.	Fasciotomy incisions and open muscle masses may be distressing to patient to see if need for fasciotomy and frequent dressing changes is not clear to patient or family.
Prepare patient for return to operating suite for split-thickness skin grafts, if done.	Split-thickness skin grafts are often needed to close large fascial defects to avoid constricting or binding scar tissue from developing if fascia is pulled too tightly for closure.

Nursing Interventions	Rationales
Seek consultation with physical therapists for active or passive exercises as prescribed.	Exercises help patient retain some muscle strength while recovering from injury.

DISCHARGE PLANNING/CONTINUITY OF CARE

- Refer to home care nurses for follow-up wound care.
- Refer to physical therapist for active range-of-motion and strengthening exercises.
- Secure appointment for return to physician.

REFERENCES

Ross, D. (1991). Acute compartment syndrome. *Orthopaedic Nursing, 10*(2), 33–38.

VOLKMANN ISCHEMIC CONTRACTURE

Volkmann ischemic contracture is a severe deformity and muscle contracture that develops secondary to unrelieved elevation of venous pressures leading to decreased arterial perfusion causing tissue ischemia, leading to death of cells. The cells that die are eventually replaced with scar tissue. A permanent contracture develops producing a "claw" hand or foot with markedly flexed fingers or toes and hard, leathery skin.

ETIOLOGIES

- Prolonged, unrelieved, increased venous pressures in injured tissues
- Decreased arterial perfusion
- Tissue eschemia lasting 6–12 h

CLINICAL MANIFESTATIONS

- Marked edema of injured tissues
- Marked increase in pain with passive movement of tissues
- Scar tissue formation with development of contracture(s)

CLINICAL/DIAGNOSTIC FINDINGS

- Electromyogram (EMG) studies showing marked decrease or absent muscle/nerve response to stimuli
- Physical examination showing contracture(s) of digits or toes, wrist, elbow, or ankle joint, with edema
- Hard, leathery skin or marked edema of digits or toes
- Presence of fasciotomy scars

▶ NURSING DIAGNOSIS: *Body Image Disturbance*

Related To presence of nonfunctional limb and claw fingers or toes

Defining Characteristics

- Withdrawal from usual social relationships
- States is right handed and now cannot use right hand or arm
- Keeps glove on hand and wears long-sleeved clothing
- Asks if function is permanently lost

Patient Outcomes

The patient will

- participate in prescribed treatment regimen.
- develop positive social relationship over time.
- regain partial use of fingers after treatments.

Nursing Interventions	Rationales
Assess affected limb/fingers/toes for skin condition and remaining functions.	Assessment of present status of affected limb is necessary to develop specific care plans.
Seek consultation with physical therapists for prescribed exercises and other therapies.	Specific active-assisted or passive-assisted exercises help regain or retain muscular functions, if possible.
Seek consultation with occupational therapists for personal and home management techniques if necessary.	Occupational therapists assist with learning to use remaining strengths to do activities of daily living (ADL) as able, to do home management skills, and to learn how to use limb for writing or other skills as able.
Prepare patient for diagnostic tests.	More than one EMG may be done over time to determine effects of treatments.
Prepare for surgical repairs, if done.	Surgical treatments may involve tendon transplants, joint arthrodesis, or other procedures to make limb/hand/toes more "functional" with the remaining tissues.
Allow patient/family members to verbalize feelings or concerns related to deformed or useless limb/hand/foot or other tissues.	Verbalizations vary with the stage of grieving of the patient or family members, who may or may not be at similar stages or have similar feelings.

Nursing Interventions	Rationales
Seek consultation with social workers or mental health personnel as needed.	Specialists in communication skills and handling vocational/educational/financial concerns help adjustments related to the limitations that affected limb may have on the patient's return to social, familial, employment, or financial roles.
Encourage active participation in treatment regimen.	Encouragement may be vital to help the patient remain positive due to very slow, almost imperceptible changes as functions are partially regained after treatments and surgery.

NOTE: The nursing diagnoses, patient outcomes, and interventions and rationales associated with compartment syndrome (page 299) are all pertinent and vital to prevent Volkmann ischemic contracture, which will cause life-long changes and adjustments if it occurs.

DISCHARGE PLANNING/CONTINUITY OF CARE

- Refer to rehabilitation physician for long-term care.
- Refer to physical therapist for active exercises.
- Refer to occupational therapist for splints and home and employment concerns.
- Make return-to-physician appointment.

REFERENCES

Lapuk, S., & Woodbury, D. F. (1988). Volkmann ischemic contracture, a case report. *Orthopaedic Review, 17*(6), 618–624.

Mabee, J. R., & Bostwick, T. L. (1993). Pathophysiology and mechanisms of compartment syndrome. *Orthopaedic Review, 22*(2), 175–179.

Mourad, L. A. (1994). Alterations in musculoskeletel function. In K. L. McCance & S. E. Huether, *Pathophysiology* (2nd ed.). St. Louis: Mosby-Yearbook.

Peck, S. (1990). Crush syndrome: Pathophysiology and management. *Orthopaedic Nursing, 9*(3), 33–40.

Ross, D. (1991). Acute compartment syndrome. *Orthopaedic Nursing, 10*(2), 33–38.

Salmond, S. W., Mooney, N. E., & Verdisco, L. A. (1991). *Core curriculum for orthopaedic nursing* (2nd ed.). Pitman, NJ: Janetti.

THROMBOPHLEBITIS AND PULMONARY EMBOLISM FOLLOWING SURGERY

Thromboembolic conditions are related to venous status. Generally accepted as the main factors in the generation of venous thrombi are Virchow's triad of hypercoagulability, venous stasis, and endothelial damage (Carroll, 1993). Patients having total hip replacement have a high incidence of deep-vein thrombosis (DVT) because their surgical conditions allow these factors to occur simultaneously. Thrombi can develop via the intrinsic or extrinsic pathways of coagulation. In the intrinsic pathway, tissue thromboplastin is released from bone and soft tissue during surgical dissection, this release being reflected by the partial thromboplastin time (PTT). The extrinsic system, noted by the prothrombin time (PT), is activated by exposure of venous subendothelial collagen and subsequent platelet activation, leading to thrombin formation and the development of a fibrin clot. Hypercoagulability occurs when coagulation exceeds fibrinolysis, which occurs during reaming of the acetabulum, preparation of the femur, and impaction of the prosthesis (Paiement, et al., 1989).

ETIOLOGIES

- See Table 33.1, page 313, for risk factors
- Virchow's triad: venous stasis, vessel damage, and coagulation abnormalities

CLINICAL MANIFESTATIONS

- Edema of affected leg
- No symptoms of pain in either leg
- Tenderness or pain in calf of leg

CLINICAL/DIAGNOSTIC FINDINGS

- Contrast venogram revealing thrombus in deep saphenous vein
- Duplex imaging (a combination of ultrasound and Doppler scan) revealing thrombus in femoropopliteal vein
- Impedance plethysmography revealing thrombus in femoral vein
- Physical examination revealing marked edema of operative leg and thigh

▶ NURSING DIAGNOSIS: *High Risk for Pulmonary Embolism and Potential for Impaired Gas Exchange*

Risk Factors

- Postoperative patient after total hip replacement revision
- 70 years of age
- Thrombus in femoropopliteal vein

Patient Outcomes

The patient will

- not develop a pulmonary embolism.
- not develop fat emboli.
- receive prophylactic medications to prevent thromboembolism.

Nursing Interventions	Rationales
Assess patient for presence of risk factors listed in Table 33.1, page 313.	After a revision total hip replacement, the patient will have moderate tissue trauma in the operative limb, and will be on bedrest from 1–3 days, requiring skilled nursing care to prevent formation of thrombi.
Observe operative limb for edema and compare with opposite limb.	The operative limb may have moderate edema, even with leg-to-thigh wrappings or thigh-high anti-embolism hose.
Listen for patient's complaint of calf or thigh tenderness or soreness in response to nurse's question.	Tenderness or dull, aching pain in the saphenous vein in the calf or the femoropopliteal vein in the thigh may indicate the presence of thrombi in the venous system.
Perform Homan check of calf.	Homan check is dorsiflexion of the foot toward the calf. Positive result may indicate a thrombus in

Nursing Interventions	Rationales
	the saphenous, tibial, peroneal, popliteal, or common femoral veins.
Apply prescribed external compressive pneumatic garments.	These garments provide intermittent compression to the veins to lessen venous stasis.
Administer prescribed antithrombotic medications.	No one medication is used universally by all orthopaedic surgeons (see Table 33.2, page 314).
Reposition patient q2–3h.	Repositioning increases circulation to lessen venous stasis.
Listen to patient's complaints of chest pain, shortness of breath, dyspnea, anxiety, change in sensorium or level of consciousness, and confusion; access color changes.	These signs and symptoms may indicate a pulmonary embolism or cerebral embolism secondary to a peripheral or proximal (in thigh, pelvis, or heart) venous thrombus. Many of those signs may also indicate a fat embolism that can occur in older persons after hip fractures or total hip arthroplasty, believed to result from either fat particles and bone marrow forced into circulation at the time of prosthetic stem insertion and/or polymethylmethacrylate (PMMA). The use of PMMA in total joint arthroplasty has been associated with hypotension secondary to vasodilation from the residual monomer (Comadoll, Gustilio, & Rockwold, 1991). (See Table 33.3, page 315 for comparison of signs of pulmonary and fat embolisms). However, both DVT and pulmonary embolism are frequently asymptomatic; they may go undetected until major, even fatal, pulmonary embolism occurs (Roberts et al., 1989).

Nursing Interventions	Rationales
Monitor results of postoperative noninvasive or invasive studies to detect DVT.	Studies may include impedance plethysmography, ultrasound, platelet scanning, venogram, or pre- and postoperative venograms.
Monitor results of PTT or PT.	Partial thromboplastin times are done for patients receiving heparin, while PTs are done for those receiving warfarin (coumadin).
Explain purposes of multiple diagnostic or therapeutic examinations to patient and family members.	Examinations are tiring and time consuming and require cooperation from the patient. Learning of the value of the specific examination is beneficial to the patient.
Teach patient of signs and symptoms to report to physician prior to discharge.	Because of cost containment and diagnostic-related groupings (DRGs), patients following total hip arthroplasties are being discharged approximately 5 days postoperatively. Patients may develop DVTs as late as 14–21 days postoperatively and precipitous pulmonary embolism can form 1–3 weeks postoperatively (Mallory, Vaughn, Lombardi, & Mitchell, 1990).
Provide nursing care according to prescribed treatments in the event of development of fat or pulmonary embolism. See treatments listed in Table 33.3, page 315.	

DISCHARGE PLANNING/CONTINUITY OF CARE

- Refer to home care nurses for follow-up evaluation of affected leg(s), application of antithrombotic hose, and assistance with activities of daily living as needed.
- Review signs or symptoms to notify physician if they occur: increased pain, edema, soreness in legs, chest pain, shortness of breath, dyspnea, or pain on inspiration.
- Secure return-to-physician appointment.

Clinical Clip

Thromboembolic disease is a major public health problem in North America, with an estimated 200,000 people who die each year of pulmonary embolism (Paiement et al., 1989). More than 50% of these patients die in modern general hospitals while under the care of competent physicians (Paiement et al., 1989).

Total joint replacement surgeries carry a heightened risk of venous thromboembolism due to the risk factors listed in Table 33.1, page 313 (Paiement et al., 1989). Thromboembolism is responsible for 50% of postoperative mortalities in the first 3 months after hip arthroplasty (Comadoll et al., 1991).

Clinical Clip

The concept of using some form of prophylaxis to prevent the development of DVT and pulmonary embolism following total hip replacement and total knee replacement is now well accepted by orthopaedic surgeons. Ninety-six percent of orthopaedic surgeons now use some form of prophylaxis against thromboembolism following total hip or total knee replacement (Wilde, Colwell, Paiement, Pellegrini, Salvati, & Stulberg, 1993).

Clinical Clip

The incidence of DVT following total hip replacement without prophylaxis is 50% and after total knee replacement without prophylaxis it has been reported to be 70% (Wilde, et al., 1993).

Table 33.1 • Risk Factors in Postoperative Thromboembolism

Operations in the lower extremities or pelvis
Tissue trauma
Immobility
Age, over 40 years
History of previous thromboembolism
Varicose veins
Congestive heart failure
Malignant tumors

Table 33.1 • *continued*

Obesity
Increased blood viscosity
Oral contraceptive use
Inherited factors
Sepsis
Fractures
Pregnancy

Table 33.2 • Methods Used for Preventing Deep-Vein Thrombosis

Aspirin
  For men only*
  For both men and women

Warfarin (coumadin)
Heparin, dosage according to PTT
Low-dose heparin
Low-molecular-weight heparin
Dextran
Dihydroergotamine
External pneumatic compression
Compression stockings
Vena cava filter
Ambulation
Continuous passive motion

**Studies of the anticoagulant effects of aspirin have only been completed on men; women studies are now underway.*

Table 33.3 • Comparisons of Fat and Pulmonary Emboli

	Fat Emboli	Pulmonary Emboli
Pathophysiology	Emboli develop as a result of release of fat molecules from marrow of fractured long bones into bloodstream or from chemical changes in the blood following trauma; there may be multiple microemboli or large emboli that obstruct pulmonary circulation and circulation in other organs	Emboli develop secondary to thrombophlebitis; they become dislodged, travel in the bloodstream through the heart, and become lodged in the pulmonary circulation, causing obstruction
Occurrence	Most frequently 1–3 days after a long-bone fracture but can also occur at later periods	Frequently 7–10 days after trauma or development of thrombophlebitis, though can occur weeks or months later
Signs/ symptoms	Sudden development of shortness of breath and dyspnea, changes in mental alertness, confusion, sense of danger, tachycardia, tachypnea, chest pain, drop in blood pressure and appearance of fine, petechial rash from nipple line on chest, up to neck, and on eyelids or conjunctivae, pallor, or cyanosis	Same as for fat emboli, except for rash
Diagnosis	History of long-bone fracture; physical examination with presence of petechiae over chest, neck, and conjunctivae; chest x-ray; arterial blood gases (PaO_2 below 60 mm Hg); postoperative total hip arthroplasty	History of thrombophlebitis; physical examination; arterial blood gases; complete blood count with differential; ventilation and perfusion scans; chest x-ray; pulmonary angiography

Table 33.3 • *continued*

	Fat Emboli	Pulmonary Emboli
Treatments	Bed rest, O_2 therapy, mechanical ventilation if needed, external hypothermia if hyper-pyrexic, administration of steroids, heparin therapy, intravenous alcohol, administration of antibi-otics, intravenous albumin, intravenous hypertonic glucose with insulin coverage	Bed rest, O_2 therapy, intravenous heparin therapy, antibiotic administration, long-term administration of anti-coagulant medications

Source: From The nursing process in the care of adults with orthopaedic condi-tions, *3rd ed., by Mourad, L. A. and Droste, M. M., 1993, Albany, NY: Delmar. Reprinted by permission.*

REFERENCES

Barnes, C. L., Nelson, C. L., & McCowan, T. C. (1991). Preoperative venography. *Orthopaedic Review, 20*(9), 763–766.

Carroll, P. (1993). Deep venous thrombosis: Implications for orthopaedic nursing. *Orthopaedic Nursing, 12*(3), 33–42.

Comadoll, J. L., Gustilio, R. B., & Rockwold, G. L. (1991). Symptomatic intracranial meningiomas after total joint replacement. *Orthopedics, 14*(3), 347–351.

Grossman, R. S. (1993). Changing patterns of prophylaxis for deep venous thrombosis following elective hip replacement. *Orthopedics, 16*(1), 19–22.

Mallory, T. H., Vaughn, B. K., Lombardi, A. V. Jr., & Mitchell, M. (1990). Impedance plethysmography for surveillance of deep venous thrombosis following early discharge of total joint replacement patients. *Orthopedics, 13*(12), 1347–1351.

Mourad, L. A., & Droste, M. M. (1993). *The nursing process in the care of adults with orthopaedic conditions* (3rd ed.). Albany: Delmar.

Paiement, G. D., Beisaw, N., Lotke, P. A., Elia, E. A., Wessinger, S. A., & Harris, W. H. (1989). Advances in the prevention of venous thromboembolic disease after hip and knee surgery. *Orthopaedic Review, 18*(Suppl.), 1–20.

Robert, J. H., Hoffmeyer, P., Broquet, P. E., & Cerutti, P., & Vasey, H. (1993). Fat embolism syndrome. *Orthopaedic Review, 22*(5), 567–571.

Roberts, T. S., Nelson, C. L., Barnes, C. L., Boone, D. W., Ferris, E. J., & Holder, J. L. (1989). Low dose dextran 40 in reconstructive hip surgery patients. *Orthopedics, 12*(6), 797–801.

Siegel, R. S., Rae, J. L., Ryan, N. L., Edwards, C., Fortune, W. P., Lewis, R. J., & Reba, R. C. (1989). The use of indium-111 labeled platelet scanning for the detection of asymptomatic deep venous thrombosis in a high risk population. *Orthopedics, 12*(11), 1439–1443.

Wilde, A. H. (Moderator), Colwell, C. W., Paiement, G., Pellegrini, V. D., Salvati, E. A., & Stulberg, B. N. (1993). Symposium: Advances in the prevention of venous thromboembolic disease in orthopaedics: The introduction of LMWH. *Contemporary Orthopaedics, 27*(6), 551–577.

AVASCULAR NECROSIS

Avascular necrosis (AVN) or osteonecrosis can be a primary condition of bone or a secondary one as a complication following ischemia to a bone. Primary avascular necrosis is related to the risk factors of trauma, caisson disease, use of systemic steroids, alcohol abuse, radiation, connective tissue disease, sickle cell disease, and unknown cause (Childs, 1993; Safran, 1993). Secondary AVN develops after treatment with hip nails or pins for repairing fractures of the femoral neck or after treatments in younger persons with slipped capital epiphyses for Legg-Calve-Perthes disease. The AVN may involve any bone, but most commonly, the femoral head is involved, either unilaterally or bilaterally. Other bones that may develop AVN include the tarsal navicular bone (referred to as Kohler disease) and the navicular or lunate bones of the wrist (referred to as Kienbock disease).

Avascular necrosis may develop after an ischemic episode in the microcirculation of a bone or after a chronic process that alters the venous or arterial circulation to that bone, such as compartment syndrome, decompression syndrome (caisson disease), and Raynaud phenomenon. Also, whenever occlusive processes such as arteriosclerosis, sickle cell disease or fat emboli cause ischemic necrosis, AVN can develop, secondary to the rise in intraosseous pressures. Fat globules are believed to block venous outflow, causing both inflow and outflow congestion, producing edema and ischemia (Chang, Greenspan, & Gershwin, 1993; Childs, 1993). Regardless of the cause, the microcirculation of the bone is affected with the development of AVN, as the result of ischemia or decreased circulation.

Avascular necrosis results in the collapse of the "architecture" of the affected bone—with flattening or deformity of the bone leading to pain or subluxation or dislocation of the bone from the joint in severe cases—and affects joint function and mobility.

ETIOLOGIES

- Alcohol abuse
- Caisson (decompression) disease
- Cigarette smoking
- Fat emboli
- Gout
- Radiation therapy
- Raynaud phenomenon
- Sickle cell disease with increased blood viscosity
- Systemic steroids

- Trauma, such as fracture, disrupting circulation in the bone
- Unknown cause, known as idiopathic AVN

CLINICAL MANIFESTATIONS

- Arteriovenous spasms, as with Raynaud phenomenon
- Joint deformity and change in range-of-motion (ROM)
- Acute pain, with or without weight bearing, with radiation to contiguous areas
- Weakness of affected bone/joint

CLINICAL/DIAGNOSTIC FINDINGS

- Core biopsy revealing cellular bone/cartilage changes
- Computerized tomography (CT) scan and magnetic resonance imaging (MRI) revealing AVN areas and stage in involved bone(s)
- History of trauma to one or more bones
- Intramedullary pressure readings >30 mm Hg (normal is 20 mm Hg) (Childs, 1993)
- Physical examination revealing joint deformity, pain on palpation of affected bone, with radiation, at times, to contiguous areas
- Roentgenograms that may be negative initially, but, over time, show areas of joint surface collapse, deformity in normal bone anatomy, and osteoarthritic changes

▶ NURSING DIAGNOSIS: *Impaired Physical Mobility*

Related To AVN of femoral head or tarsal navicular bone

Defining Characteristics

- Joint deformity
- Limitation of movement
- Limp
- Pain in foot (tarsal navicular) or in hip, thigh or buttocks area (femoral head)

Patient Outcomes

The patient will

- experience relief of pain and limp with treatments.
- have no additional AVN in other bones.

Nursing Interventions	Rationales
Assess symptoms of pain and limp: when occurs; severity, duration, and relief measures used; and results of relief measures.	Patient data determine basis for care.

Nursing Interventions	Rationales
Discuss medical plan of care, after physician's explanations.	Repeated explanations or clarifications may be required because of anxiety or newness of diagnosis.
Provide crutches, if prescribed; apply shoulder pads, wrist pads, and rubber tips to crutches.	Use of crutches for 6 months or longer protects the affected bone/joint from weight-bearing stresses. The pads and tips on crutches provide safety for their use.
Seek consultation with physical therapist for prescribed exercises.	Exercises help maintain strength and ROM to involved muscles and joints.
Teach patient proper crutch walking techniques.	The patient will need instruction about amount of weight bearing allowed, techniques for ascending and descending stairs, and sitting and rising from chairs.
Teach patient purposes of pulsed electromagnetic fields (PEMFs), if used.	Pulsed electromagnetic fields provide pulses of electrical energy to cells of the affected bone, on the theory that bone growth is stimulated by increased osteoblastic activity (osteoblasts are bone-forming cells), leading to revascularization of affected ischemic bone. Electric pulses are directed to the bone through coils held on the skin with velcro straps. It is a painless treatment.

▶ NURSING DIAGNOSIS: *Acute Pain*

Related To ischemic changes and degeneration of involved bone

Defining Characteristics

- Limp due to pain
- Pain with weight bearing, at times when non–weight bearing, and sometimes at night
- Radiation of pain to heel or top of foot (if navicular bone involved) or to thigh, buttocks, or knee (if femoral head involved)

Patient Outcomes

The patient will

- be relieved of pain with analgesics and other treatments.
- experience relief of AVN.

Nursing Interventions	Rationales
Assess pain characteristics, sites, severity, and duration.	Patient's pain may or may not be related to weight bearing. It may radiate to contiguous areas and may vary from dull to sharp.
Administer prescribed analgesics and/or anti-inflammatory medications.	Analgesics relieve the acute pain when administered at therapeutic levels and at required intervals. Anti-inflammatory medications relieve the pathology related to the AVN, thereby also relieving pain.
Discuss use of crutches, exercises, and PEMFs, as under previous nursing diagnosis.	Use of these treatments also provides pain relief.
Discuss surgical corrective procedure (rotational osteotomy or core decompression) after physician's explanation.	Surgical procedures consist of rotational osteotomy, which involves displacing the avascular necrotic segment out of the weight-bearing region in favor of intact overlying cartilage (Safran, 1993). It reduces stress on the bone during healing so it does not collapse. During rotational osteotomy, the head of the femur is rotated so that a normal posterior portion is placed in the weight-bearing zone. The cut bone areas are held together with internal fixation plates and screws. This operation does not always stop the AVN or the progression of osteoarthritis, if present (Safran, 1993). Core decompression of the head of the femur, along with placement of a bone graft or bone plug to the area of decompression, is done on

Nursing Interventions	Rationales
	the theory that revascularization will provide a stable fusion with existing bone and halt the bone necrosis (Childs, 1993).
	Eventually, a total joint replacement may need to be done, as discussed in Chapters 19–21, or a joint fusion.

DISCHARGE PLANNING/CONTINUITY OF CARE

- Refer to home care nurses for evaluation of wound healing, ambulation, and nutritional assistance, as needed.
- Refer to physical therapy for ROM exercises.
- Make return-to-physician appointment.
- Review prescribed medication regimen and side effects of medications.

REFERENCES

Chang, C. C., Greenspan, A., & Gershwin, M. E. (1993). Osteonecrosis: Current perspectives on pathogenesis and treatments. *Seminars in Arthritis and Rheumatism, 23*(1), 47–69.

Childs, S. (1993). Avascular necrosis of the bone: The causes and the cures. *Orthopaedic Nursing, 12*(4), 29–34.

Safran M. R. (1993). Rotational osteotomy buys time on AVN of femoral head. *Orthopedics Today, 12*(11), 22.

BONE UNION PROBLEMS

After injury to a bone that results in a fracture, the bone healing process may lead to complicated union problems such as the following:

- *Delayed union:* prolonged period before evidence of callus formation is noted; usually referred to as delayed after 5–7 months, depending on the type of fracture and bone involved
- *Joint fusion:* bone union and joint structures that heal with stiffness or rigidity (fusion) if the injury or fracture was through or within a joint
- *Malunion:* nonanatomic union or healing of bone
- *Nonunion:* failure to develop callus at a fracture site; usually not declared a nonunion until 7–9 months or longer after a fracture
- *Pseudarthrosis:* "false" joint forming at or near site of the original fracture
- *Refracture:* recurrence of a fracture at site of original fracture

ETIOLOGIES

- Corticosteroid administration, long term
- Decreased circulation to area of fracture
- Diabetes
- Inadequate immobilization
- Infection
- Interposed soft tissue between fracture ends of bone
- Malignant tumor at site
- Malnutrition
- Systemic inflammatory disease, as, e.g., rheumatoid arthritis
- Too much bone loss
- Too rigid immobilization

CLINICAL MANIFESTATIONS

- Decreased range of motion (ROM)
- Deformity of bone
- Inability to bear weight
- Movement at site
- Pain with use or weight bearing
- Stiffness of joint

CLINICAL/DIAGNOSTIC FINDINGS

- History of past injury with fracture
- Magnetic resonance imaging (MRI) or computerized tomography (CT) scan revealing soft tissue interposed between fracture ends of bone
- Physical examination revealing abnormal movement at site of fracture, malunion, pain, tenderness, decreased ROM, and inability to use or bear weight properly
- Roentgenograms revealing lack of callus formation

▶ NURSING DIAGNOSIS: *Acute Pain*

Related To nonunion, malunion, or delayed union.

Defining Characteristics

- Awakens at night with pain
- Has pain with use

Patient Outcomes

The patient will

- experience healing of fracture site with adequate callus.
- experience relief of pain with medications and other treatments.

Nursing Interventions	Rationales
Assess characteristics, duration, and severity of pain.	Data are vital for individualized care.
Position patient for comfort; use pillows as necessary.	Presence of pain may interfere with positioning. Pillows provide a softer surface for extremity.
Elevate extremity; if upper extremity, place in sling.	Elevation decreases edema formation to decrease pressure on nerve endings and thereby decrease pain.
Administer analgesics as prescribed.	Analgesics decrease perception of pain.
Support the joints above and below the affected area when lifting or moving extremity.	Support under the joints rather than under soft tissues prevents additional injury through moving the muscles and joints, which puts pressure on the unhealed bone.

▶ NURSING DIAGNOSIS: *Impaired Physical Mobility*

Related To nonunion or pseudarthrosis

Defining Characteristics

- MRI evidence of soft tissue interposed between ends of fractured bones
- Roentgen evidence of lack of callus at fracture site

Patient Outcomes

The patient will have:

- no soft tissue between fractured bone ends.
- well-healed, callus formation at fracture site with treatments.

Nursing Interventions	Rationales
Assess fracture site for open areas, edema, deformity, color, and temperature.	These signs or symptoms are all related to fracture healing and the inflammatory process.
Observe patient's use of crutches or walker or application of sling if upper extremity.	The patient will have used crutches for 7–9 months and so should be proficient but may have developed some poor techniques that need correcting.
Determine how much weight is being put on affected extremity.	The patient may be allowed partial weight bearing.
Prepare the patient for open exploration and application of compression plate and screws or placement of bone grafts to site.	A nonunion or pseudarthrosis will require open reduction and fixation for healing to occur. Removal of the interposed tissue should allow approximation of fractured bone ends for healing and callus formation.
Clarify bone-healing processes with patient and family members.	The patient may not be fully aware that the fracture site will be treated as if it is a "fresh" fracture. (See Table 1.3, page 19 for stages of fracture healing).
Perform all nine neurovascular checks every hour initially, then as prescribed.	Because of open surgery, the extremity must be closely observed to prevent development of compartment syndrome, hemorrhage, or wound infection.

Nursing Interventions	Rationales
Teach patient wound care prior to discharge; provide written instructions.	Being able to do self-care is positive for patients and provides safety to prevent infection.
Teach patient steps of neurovascular checks and how to do each check. Provide written instructions.	Understanding purposes of checks helps patient do self-care safely and to note changes if they occur.
Complete continuity-of-care referral.	Referral permits care to continue after discharge.

DISCHARGE PLANNING/CONTINUITY OF CARE

- Make return-to-physician appointment.
- Referral to home care nurses for evaluation of use of crutches, and ambulation.
- Provide a written list of neurovascular checks.

REFERENCES

Barnes, C. L., Nix, M. L., Lavender, R. C., & Nelson, C. L. (1991). Duplex scanning in orthopaedic patients. *Contemporary Orthopaedics, 22*(3), 283–286.

HETEROTOPIC OSSIFICATION (MYOSITIS OSSIFICANS TRAUMATICA OR MYOSITIS OSSIFICANS CIRCUMSCRIPTA)

Myositis ossificans circumscripta (MOC) occurs in variable incidence according to the site and injury. It occurs in as many as two-thirds of patients undergoing acetabular open reduction and internal fixation, and after total hip arthroplasty, the incidence is reportedly 8–71%, with 2–7% of patients developing significant or symptomatic heterotopic bone (Pittenger, 1991; Warren, 1991).

ETIOLOGIES

- Burns
- Hematoma formations
- Male sex: 3 : 1 male-to-female ratio (Warren, 1991)
- Multiple sclerosis and ankylosing spondylitis
- Neurologic injuries
- Surgery, especially total hip replacement (THR)
- Trauma

CLINICAL MANIFESTATIONS

- Decreased range of motion (ROM), both actively and passively
- Erythema
- Induration (firmness or hardness)
- Pain and tenderness, usually becoming persistent pain
- Palpable mass
- Swelling at site

CLINICAL/DIAGNOSTIC FINDINGS

- Computerized tomography (CT) scan to assess extent of mass and involvement of joint
- Decrease in serum calcium levels
- Positive bone scan
- Rise in serum alkaline phosphatase levels
- Roentgenograms revealing mineralization at site of heterotopic ossification

▶ NURSING DIAGNOSIS: *Impaired Physical Mobility*

Related To development of MOC and restricted joint movements

Defining Characteristics

- Status post–total joint arthroplasty
- Status posttrauma to muscle and bone

Patient Outcomes

The patient will

- regain joint ROM with treatments.
- undergo successful removal of MOC areas without recurrence.

Nursing Interventions	Rationales
Assess ROM of affected extremity and effects on mobility.	Determines severity of problem. Some patients have severely restricted ROM (Warren, 1991).
Provide crutches or walker to assist patient's ambulation.	Crutches or walker lessen stress on affected tissues to slow buildup of ossified tissues.
Administer prescribed medications such as diphosphonates, e.g., Etidronate.	Diphosphonates are used to help develop a useful joint ROM prior to mineralization of osteoid (Pittenger, 1991).
Observe for side effects of Etidronate.	Side effects include nausea and gastrointestinal upset and osteomalacia (decreased bone mineralization).
Administer indomethacin or ibuprofen, if prescribed.	Indomethacin is an anti-inflammatory medication that affects bone metabolism to help prevent development of MOC. Ibuprofen is also an

Nursing Interventions	Rationales
	anti-inflammatory medication that has been effective to prevent MOC in 50% of patients (Healy, Lo, Pfeifer, & Wasilewski, 1992).
Explain purposes and effects of radiation therapy, if given.	Radiation therapy arrests the initial step in osteoid formation by altering DNA transcription (Pittenger, 1991). Dosage varies from 2,000 to 3,000 rad over 10 doses or single-dose radiation given on first postoperative days (Healy et al., 1992; Pellegrini, Konski, Gastel, Rubin, & Evarts, 1992).
Prepare patient for surgical resection of MOC, if MOC is fully established, and above treatments not used.	Approximately 18 months are needed for ectopic bone (MOC)to have stopped growing or matured for it to be excised and not recur (Pittenger, 1991). Usual postoperative care is given after removal of the MOC lesion.

DISCHARGE PLANNING/CONTINUITY OF CARE

- Refer to home care nurses for follow-up wound care (if mass removed).
- Refer to physical therapy for diathermy and ROM exercises.
- Make return-to-physician appointment.

REFERENCES

Cushner, F. D., & Morwessel, R. M. (1992). Myositis ossificans traumatica. *Orthopaedic Review, 21*(11), 1319–1326.

Healy, W. L., Lo, T. C. M., Pfeifer, B. A., & Wasilewski, S. A. (1992). Radiotherapy in the prevention of heterotopic ossification after total hip arthroplasty. *Complications in Orthopedics, 7*(2), 207–210.

Pellegrini, V. D., Konski, A. A., Gastel, J. A., Rubin, P., & Evarts, C. McM. (1992). Prevention of heterotopic ossification with irradiation after total hip arthroplasty: Radiation therapy with a single dose of eight hundred centigray administered to a limited field. *Journal of Bone and Joint Surgery, 74-A*(2), 186–200.

Pittenger, D. E. (1991). Heterotopic ossification. *Orthopaedic Review, 20*(1), 33–39.

Warren, S. B. (1991). Heterotopic ossification after total hip replacement. *Orthopaedic Review, Dec.* (Suppl.), *20*(XX), 3–10.

INDEX

Tables are indicated by *t*

B

C

D

Q

R

S

T

U

V

W

Z